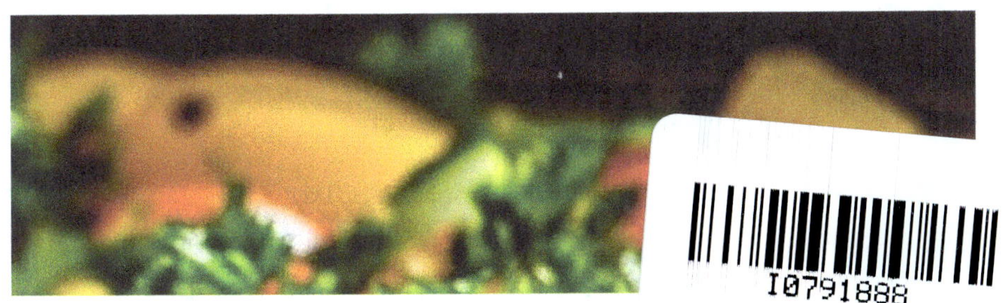

FIRE UP YOUR METABOLISM

A 30-DAY

COOKBOOK FOR WOMEN

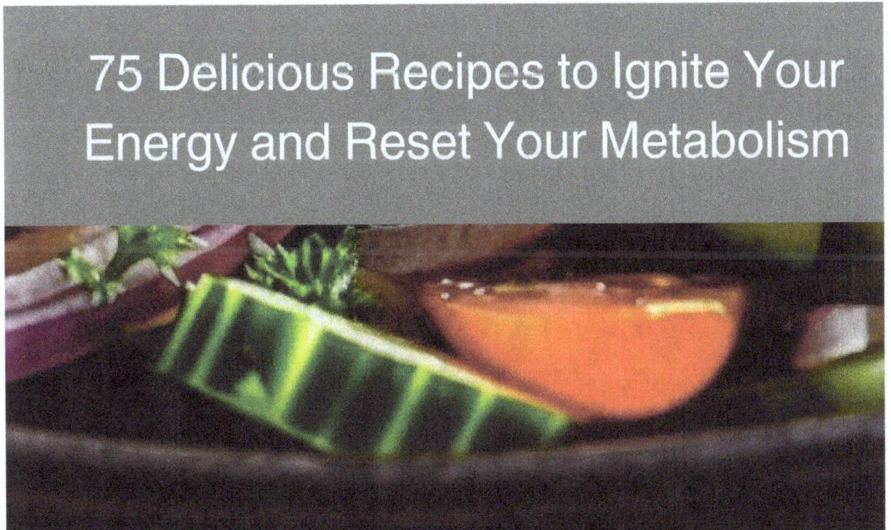

COPYRIGHT

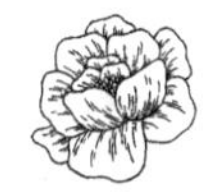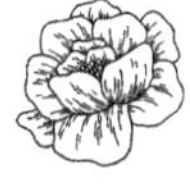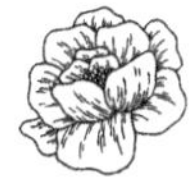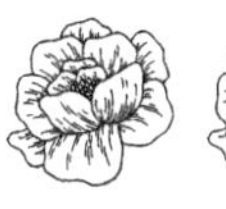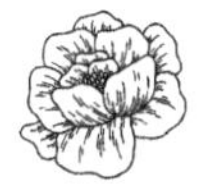

This Book is dedicated to my family

Laura, Sam, Alice and Felicia

I LOVE YOU SO MUCH

TABLE OF CONTENT

INTRODUCTION

SARAH'S JOURNEY TO METABOLISM

My adversary used to be the mirror. It was a stranger's reflection staring back, a pallid, worn-out replica of the Sarah I knew years ago. My baggy garments served as a continual reminder of the vivid vitality I had lost. My days were a haze of lazy mornings, drowsy afternoons, and nights spent longing for a glimmer of my old self.

Once a source of delight, food has turned into a combat zone. I tried everything: tight eating plans, trendy diets, and even juice fasts. They all claimed to have a magical reset, but all they offered was hopelessness and a growing sense of helplessness. It appeared as though my metabolism had turned into a lethargic engine that would not start again no matter how hard I tried.

An air of silent desperation replaced the frustration. I missed the Sarah who could run around in the park after my nephews and who got up with the sun, eager to start the day. It was while browsing a health forum that I came across the term "metabolism boosting." There was a ray of optimism in it. I threw myself into my research, watching endless videos and reading a ton of articles. Gradually a fresh viewpoint surfaced. It was about realizing my body's specific demands, not about punishing it with deprivation.

It was not an easy road. Some days, the seductive cries of pizza and ice cream were irresistible. But every mouthful of a nutrient-dense breakfast, every brisk stroll in the morning, I sensed a glimmer of change.

My energy began to increase, and that afternoon lull vanished from my mind. The mirror, which was once an adversary, now witnessed a change. The woman who was facing him had more brightness in her eyes and a more assured stance.

Though the physical improvements were a nice bonus, it wasn't just about that. It has to do with taking back my life. I regain the excitement of a solid workout and the joy of movement. I took up cooking again, not out of duty but with a renewed love and enthusiasm for feeding my body.

"Fire Up Your Metabolism," the book, is the result of that trip. It's evidence of the effectiveness of knowing your body and providing it with the correct resources for nourishment. It's a guide to rekindle your inner fire and become the vibrant, vivacious woman you were always intended to be, not just a list of recipes. Come along with me, Sarah, as we set out on our journey. Let's speed up your metabolism and unleash all of your amazing body.

UNDERSTANDING YOUR METABOLISM AS A WOMAN

There's more to a woman's metabolism than just burning calories. The intricate interplay of hormones, enzymes, and cellular mechanisms governs the production and utilization of energy. To fully unleash this powerhouse within you, you must first understand how it operates.

Women's metabolisms are intriguing subjects, and this section of "Fire Up Your Metabolism" will delve into them by looking at:

The Special Dance of Hormones: We'll talk about how thyroid, estrogen, and progesterone regulate metabolism during various phases of life, such as adolescence, menstruation, pregnancy, and menopause.

Myths About Metabolism Busted: We'll dispel the notions that are often held about metabolism, such as the notion that everyone has a constant metabolic rate or that it is feasible to burn fat in a particular location.

The Power of Food as Fuel: teaches you how to make wise decisions to maintain a healthy metabolic rate as well as how various macronutrients (protein, carbs, and fats) affect metabolism.

The Mind-Body Connection: We'll look at how your metabolism may be greatly impacted by stress, sleep, and exercise, and how to best take advantage of these effects for a healthy system.

Knowing the specific mechanisms underlying your metabolism gives you the ability to:

Boost Your vigor: Bid farewell to afternoon lulls and welcome to constant vigor all day long.

Effectively Manage Your Weight: Discover how to fuel your body for maximum health and preserve a healthy weight.

Feel More in Control: Being able to manage your metabolism gives you the ability to make wise decisions regarding your overall health and wellbeing.

There is more to this section than merely scientific justifications. It's about arming you with the information and resources you need to turn your metabolism from a mysterious force to a potent partner on your path to a more vibrant, healthy version of yourself.

REFRAMING HEALTH & EMBRACING WELLBEING FOR YOU

Many women associate the word "health" with a number on a scale or with being on a restrictive diet that makes them feel like they are missing out. However, "Fire Up Your Metabolism" is more than just this. True health, in our opinion, is a colorful tapestry made of emotional equilibrium, empowerment, and physical well-being.

You will learn how to adopt a more holistic approach to health and change your viewpoint by reading this part, which focuses on:

Nourishing Your Body: Recognizing that each body is different and requires a different diet, we will discuss the idea of bio-individuality. You will have the ability to prepare delectable meals that will boost your metabolism, nourish you from the inside out, and encourage optimum health.

Moving Your Body: Get over your fear of the gym! We'll go over various enjoyable activities to move your body, such stress-relieving dancing routines and energizing hikes in the outdoors.

Making Sleep a Priority: Learn how important good sleep is for a healthy metabolism and general wellbeing. Discover useful advice for setting up a sleeping area and practicing good sleep hygiene.

Handling Stress: We'll look at how long-term stress might interfere with your metabolism and offer helpful coping mechanisms.

30 DAYS TO A REVVED-UP METABOLISM: ROADMAP TO SUCCESS

Your secret to a boosted metabolism—the engine that powers your body and keeps you feeling your best—is this 30-day plan. Put an end to restricted schedules and fad diets. This is a voyage of transformation intended to fuel your mind, nurture your body, and maximize your metabolism.

In the upcoming 30 days, you will:

- Learn how to make mouthwatering dishes that will entice your palate and boost your metabolism for long-lasting energy.
- Discover easy ways to increase your metabolism naturally, such as stress-reduction tactics and sleep hacks.
- Learn about your body's specific requirements so that you may make decisions that will best serve your health.
- Celebrate successes and watch how you change—your energy will shoot through the roof and you'll feel more alive than ever.

This roadmap is more than just a plan; it's an empowering adventure. It's about taking control of your health and well-being, one delicious meal and mindful step at a time. Are you ready to unlock your inner fire? Let's get started!

This compelling section uses strong verbs, vivid imagery, and a conversational tone to capture the reader's attention. It emphasizes the positive outcomes, the delicious recipes, and the transformative nature of the 30-day plan, making it feel exciting and achievable.

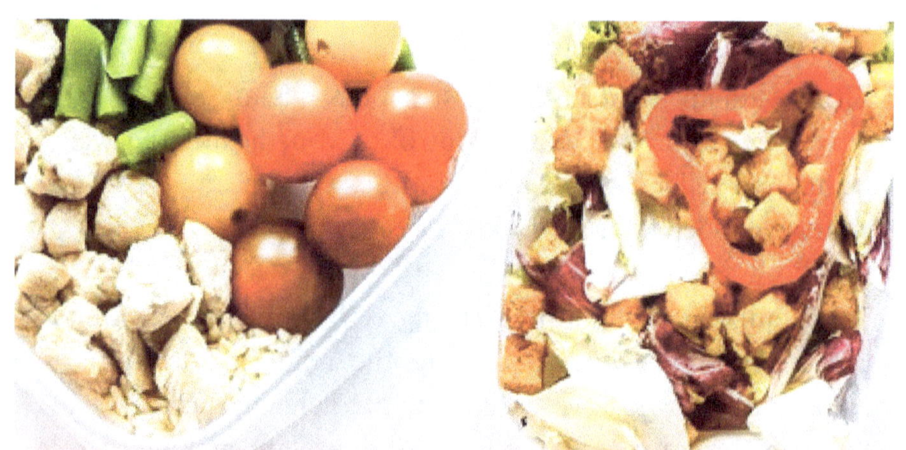

PART 1: FUELING YOUR DAY THE METABOLISM-BOOSTING WAY

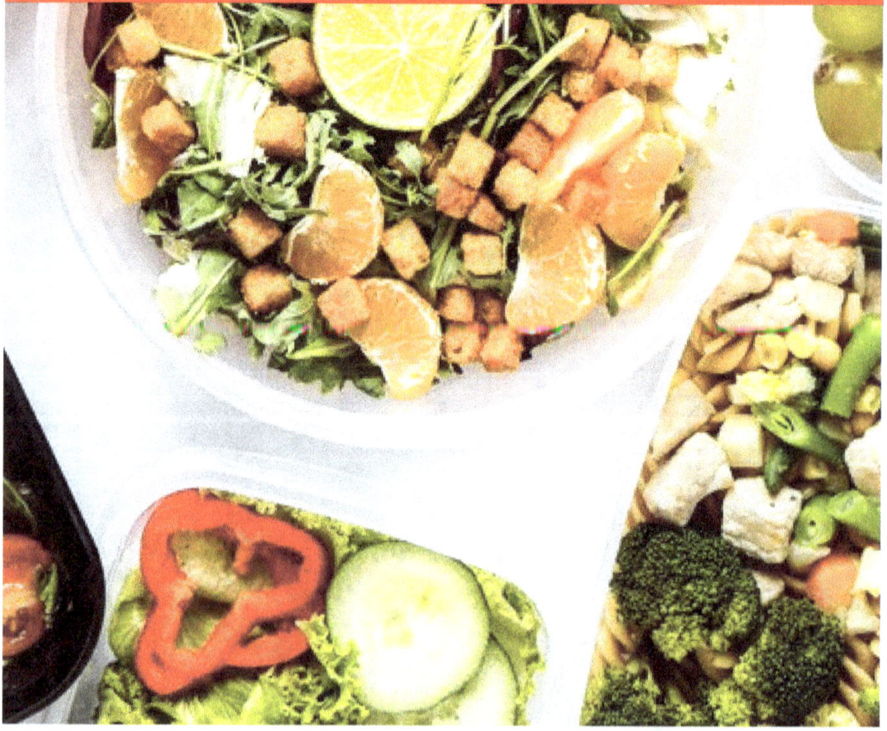

POWER UP YOUR MORNINGS - METABOLISM-MORNINGS FOR BUSY WOMEN

"You are what you eat," as the saying goes, and nowhere is this more true than with breakfast, the meal that determines how your entire day will go. Nonetheless, mornings can be a hectic jumble for working women. Choosing to hit the snooze button rather than prepare breakfast slowly is common.

This chapter is your go-to tool for handling busy mornings. We'll look at several tasty, metabolism-boosting breakfast ideas that include:

Rapid & Simple: Too busy to prepare lavish meals? Not a problem! Even the most sleep-deprived warriors can whip up a number of our dishes in a matter of minutes.

Rich in Protein: Protein is an amazing metabolic accelerator that keeps you feeling satisfied and energized all morning long. We'll demonstrate tasty and inventive ways to include foods high in protein in your morning routine.

Delicious & Filling: It doesn't have to be boring because it's healthy! Our meals will entice your taste senses and keep you full and content till noon.

Prepare to explore a world of breakfast options that will fuel your metabolism, nourish your body, and keep you feeling great all morning long—say goodbye to sugary cereals!
Let's get started!

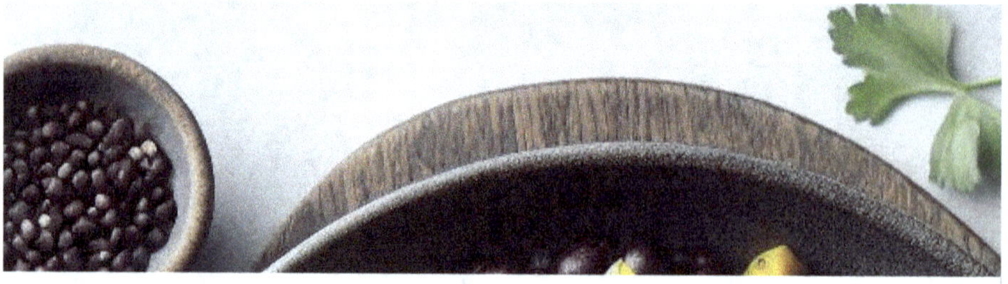

SPICY BLACK BEAN SCRAMBLE WITH AVOCADO   (Serves 1):

INGREDIENTS

- One tablespoon of olive oil
- ½ cup finely chopped onion
- ½ chopped red bell pepper
- One minced clove of garlic and ½ cup of rinsed and drained canned black beans
- Half a teaspoon of chili powder
- One-half teaspoon cumin
- A dash of cayenne (optional)
- Two big eggs
- 1/4 cup of feta cheese crumbles (optional)
- ½ sliced, ripe avocado
- To taste, add salt and pepper.

DIRECTIONS

1. In a pan set over medium heat, warm the olive oil. Saute the onion and bell pepper for five minutes, or until they become soft.
2. Once added, cook for a further minute. Add the cumin, chili powder, black beans, and cayenne (if using) and stir.
3. In the bean mixture, make two little wells, and crack an egg into each well. Add pepper and salt for seasoning.
4. Cook for 3–4 minutes, or until the yolks are cooked to your preferred consistency and the egg whites are set.
5. Add sliced avocado and crumbled feta cheese (if desired) on top.

Nutritional Information:
Calories: 350 Protein: 18g Fat: 18g
Carbs: 20g Fiber: 7g

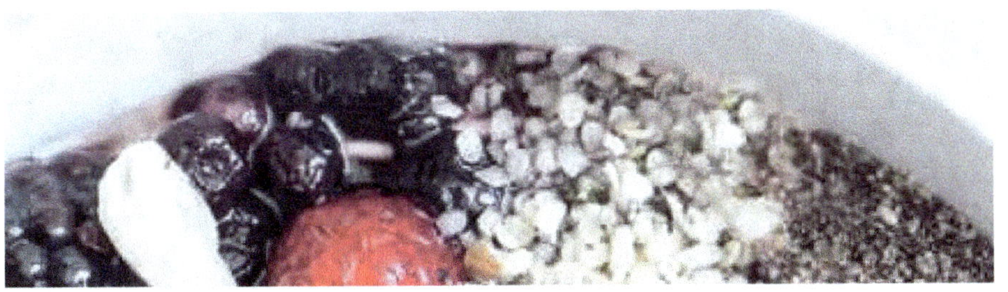

GREEK YOGURT BOWL WITH BERRIES & CHIA SEEDS (Serves 1):

INGREDIENTS

- One cup of plain Greek yogurt with a fat level of 2% or more
- ½ cup of fresh berries, such as raspberries, strawberries, and blueberries
- Two tablespoons of chia seeds
- One tablespoon of chopped nuts (pecans, walnuts, and almonds)
- A drizzle of maple syrup or honey is optional.

DIRECTIONS

1. Greek yogurt, chia seeds, and fresh berries should all be combined in a bowl.
2. Add chopped nuts and (optional) a sprinkle of honey or maple syrup on top.

Nutritional Information:

300 calories 20g of protein, 10g of fat
25g of carbohydrates   5g of fiber

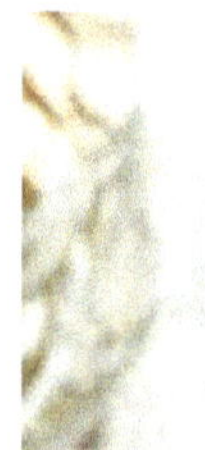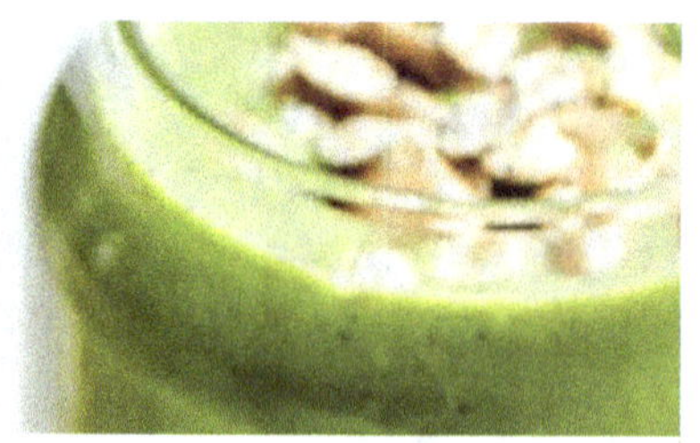

PROTEIN SMOOTHIE WITH SPINACH AND BANANA (Serves 1):

INGREDIENTS

- 1 cup almond milk without sugar
- One scoop of protein powder (chocolate or vanilla)
- ½ cup of freshly packed spinach
- 1 frozen ripe banana
- (Optional) ¼ cup plain Greek yogurt
- An optional handful of ice cubes

DIRECTIONS

1. Blend all ingredients together in a blender until smooth and creamy. Add ice cubes for a thicker consistency (optional).

Nutritional Information:
(Note: Depending on the protein powder you choose, the nutritional information may change.)
350 approximate calories   25g of protein, roughly, 10g of fat, 30g of carbs, roughly. 5g of fiber.

WHOLE-WHEAT TOAST WITH SMOKED SALMON & AVOCADO (Serves 1):

INGREDIENTS

- One slice of whole-wheat bread
- Twice as much ricotta as
- Two ounces of smoked salmon
- ½ mashed, ripe avocado
- Juice from lemons (optional)
- A pinch of optional red pepper flakes

DIRECTIONS

1. Spread some whole-wheat bread with a toast.
2. Toast with ricotta cheese spread on it.
3. Add mashed avocado and smoked salmon on top.
4. Squeeze in some lemon juice and, if desired, top with red pepper flakes.

Nutritional Information:

300 calories, 20g of protein, 15g of fat
25g of carbohydrates , 5g of fiber

SCRAMBLED EGGS WITH VEGETABLES & COTTAGE CHEESE   (Serves 1):

INGREDIENTS

- Two big eggs
- 1/4 cup finely chopped veggies (tomatoes, mushrooms, and spinach)
- 1 tablespoon finely chopped fresh herbs (dill, parsley)
- ¼ cup cottage cheese with little fat
- To taste, add salt and pepper.

DIRECTIONS

1. In a bowl, whisk together eggs, pepper, and salt.
2. A nonstick pan should be heated over medium heat. Once the veggies are softened, sauté them for two to three minutes.
3. Add the egg mixture and use a spatula to scramble until the eggs are fully cooked.
4. Before serving, fold in the cottage cheese and fresh herbs.

Nutritional Information:

Calories: 250
Protein: 22

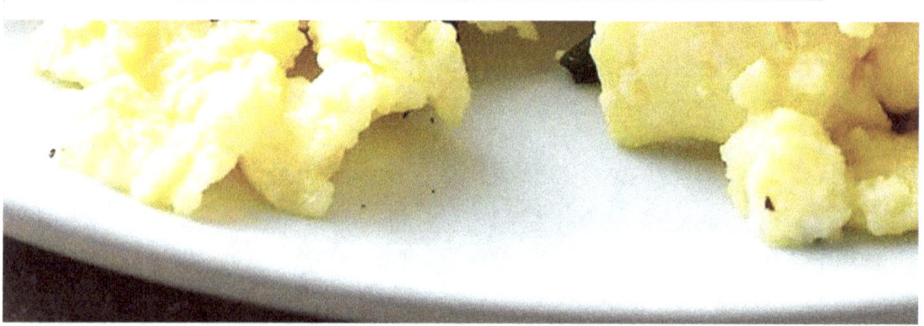

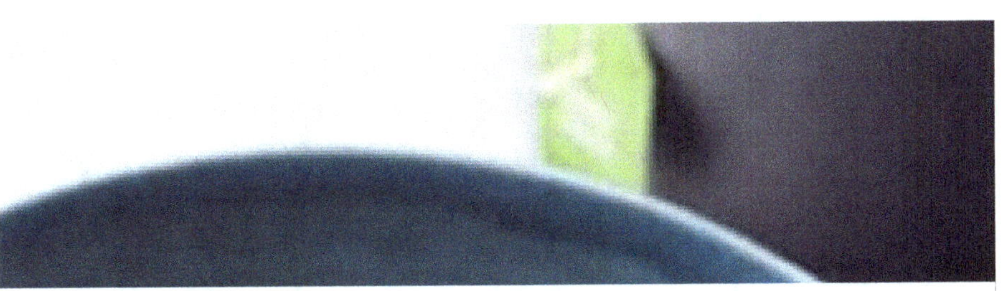

OVERNIGHT OATS WITH BERRIES AND ALMONDS   (Serves 1):

INGREDIENTS

- half a cup of rolled oats
- ½ cup almond milk without sugar
- ¼ cup of Greek yogurt, plain
- A quarter cup of berries, comprising blue, rasp, and strawberry
- 1 tsp almond slices
- 1 teaspoon of optional chia seeds
- A dash of cinnamon

DIRECTIONS

1. Rolling oats, almond milk, Greek yogurt, and chia seeds (if using) should all be combined in a jar or other container.
2. Add cinnamon and berries and stir.
3. Refrigerate the jar overnight with a lid on.
4. Top with sliced almonds and serve cold in the morning.

Nutritional Information:

320 calories, Protein (15g), Fat (12g)
35g of carbohydrates, 6g of fiber

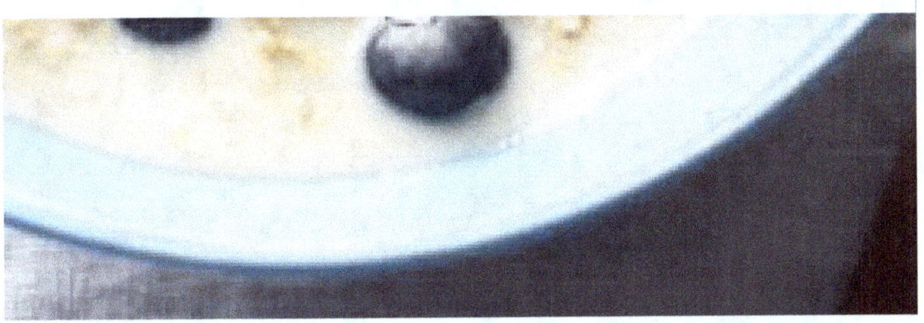

HIGH-PROTEIN BREAKFAST BURRIT

(Serves 1):

INGREDIENTS

- Single whole-wheat tortilla
- two eggs in a scramble
- 1/4 cup of washed and drained black beans
- 2 tablespoons of shredded Monterey Jack or cheddar cheese
- One tablespoon salsa (optional)
- pieces of chopped avocado (optional)

DIRECTIONS

1. In a pan, scramble two eggs. Add pepper and salt for seasoning.
2. Heat a tortilla made of whole wheat in a skillet or microwave.
3. On the tortilla, distribute the scrambled eggs.
4. Add the salsa (if using), cheese, and black beans.
5. Fold the tortilla and place optional avocado slices on top.

Nutritional Information:

350 calories, 25g of protein , 15g of fat
30g of carbohydrates, 5g of fiber

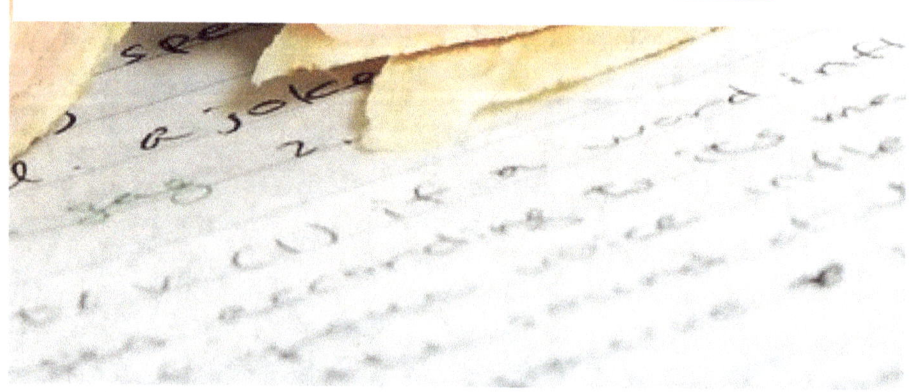

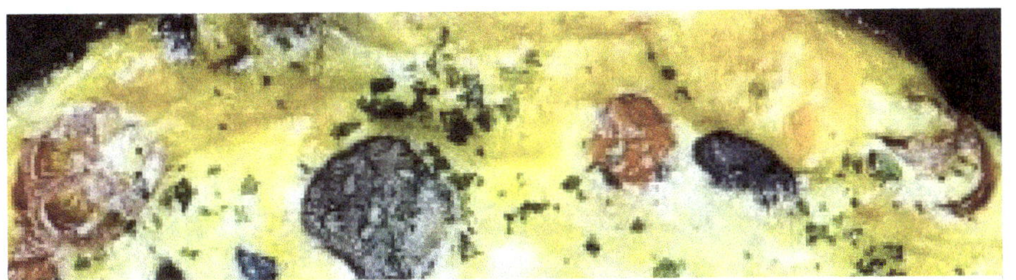

TURKEY SAUSAGE AND VEGGIE FRITTATA

(Serves 1):

INGREDIENTS

- One tablespoon of olive oil
- ½ cup of finely chopped bell peppers, onions, and broccoli
- 4 ounces of turkey sausage, ground
- Half a cup of shredded cheese (cheddar, mozzarella), beaten into six large eggs
- To taste, add salt and pepper.

Nutritional Information:

Calories: 300
Protein: 20g
Fat: 15g
Carbs: 5g
Fiber: 2g

DIRECTIONS

1. Turn the oven on to 375°F, or 190°C. Grease a small skillet that can be baked.
2. In a pan set over medium heat, warm the olive oil. Vegetables should be chopped and cooked for 5 minutes to soften them.
3. Using a spatula, break up the ground turkey sausage and sauté it until it turns brown.
4. Fill the skillet with the veggie and sausage mixture after it has been oiled.
5. Whisk the beaten eggs, salt, and pepper in a different basin.
6. Over the veggies and sausage in the skillet, pour the egg mixture.
7. Add some cheese shreds on top.
8. Bake for 20 to 25 minutes, or until the eggs are cooked through and firm in the middle.

CHIA SEED PUDDING WITH NUT BUTTER AND FRUIT   (Serves 1):

INGREDIENTS

- half a cup of chia seeds
- One cup of unsweetened plant-based milk, such as almond milk
- One tablespoon of nut butter (almond or peanut butter)
- 1/2 cup of chopped fruit (banana, berries, and mango)
- ¼ cup finely chopped nuts (walnuts, almonds)
- A drizzle of maple syrup or honey is optional.

DIRECTIONS

1. Mix the almond milk and chia seeds in a jar or other container. Give everything a good stir, then leave it for at least fifteen minutes—or overnight if you want it thicker.
2. Stir the chia pudding once more in the morning. Arrange a layer of chopped nuts, chopped fruit, and nut butter.
3. For extra sweetness, drizzle with maple syrup or honey (optional).

Nutritional Information:
300 calories, 5g of protein
15g of fat, 25g of carbohydrates
8g of fiber

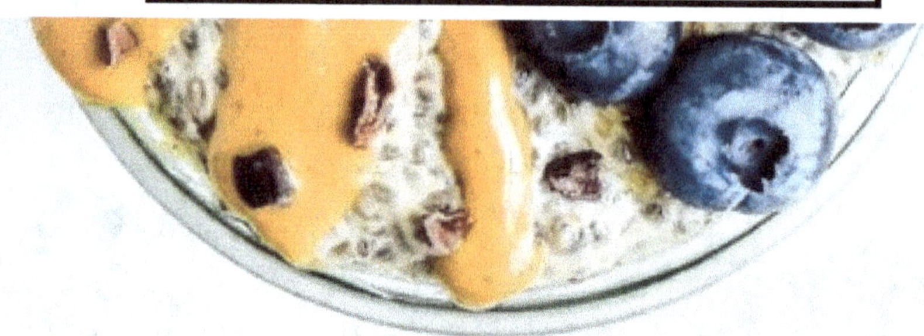

COTTAGE CHEESE PANCAKES WITH BERRIES **(Serves 1):**

INGREDIENTS

- ½ cup cottage cheese with little fat
- One big egg
- 1/2 teaspoon baking powder and 2 tablespoons whole wheat flour
- A dash of cinnamon
- berries, such as strawberries, raspberries, and blueberries
- (Optional) maple syrup

DIRECTIONS

1. Mix the cottage cheese, egg, flour, cinnamon, and baking powder in a bowl. Mix thoroughly to produce a batter.
2. Warm up a nonstick pan that has been lightly oiled over medium heat.
3. For each pancake, pour ¼ cup of batter and cook for two to three minutes on each side, or until golden brown.

Add some fresh berries on top and (optionally) sprinkle with maple syrup.

Nutritional Information:
280 calories
Protein (20g) and Fat (5g)
30g of carbohydrates
2g of fiber

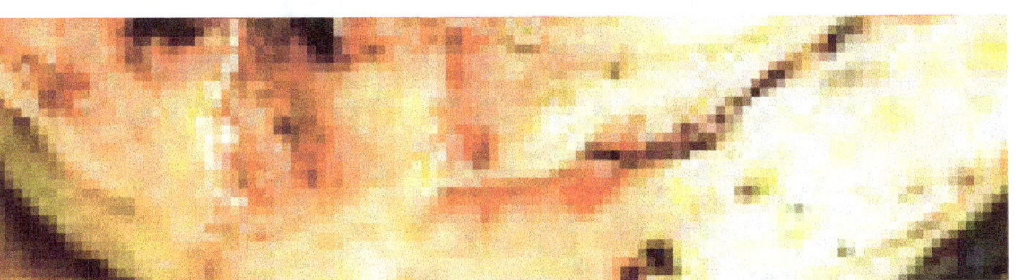

LUNCHTIME WINS – FUELING YOUR AFTERNOON WITH METABOLISM MAGIC

Beating the mornings is only the beginning of the fight. The lunchtime slump can really sap your vitality, making you seek for harmful convenience food or sugary snacks. But worry not, working women! This chapter is your go-to tactic for winning at lunch.

We'll look at several delectable and filling lunch options, like:

Perfect & Transportable: Not enough time to prepare a fancy lunch? Not a problem! We provide a selection of meals that are convenient to pack and eat on the road.

Harmonious & Invigorating: Disregard the afternoon lull! These dishes are nutrient-dense and will keep your energy levels high and your metabolism running smoothly.

Delicious & Exciting: Since being healthy shouldn't be monotonous! We provide flavor-filled dishes that will satisfy your palate and keep your body going.

Prepare to break free from the bad lunch routine and explore a plethora of delectable selections that will fuel your afternoon and maintain a high metabolism! Together, let's set out on this delectable voyage.

QUINOA SALAD WITH GRILLED CHICKEN & LEMON VINAIGRETTE (Serves 1):

INGREDIENTS

- half a cup of prepared quinoa
- Three ounces of grilled chicken breast, sliced; half a cup of chopped veggies (cherry tomatoes bell peppers, and cucumber)
- 1/4 cup of feta cheese crumbles (optional)
- Several freshly cut herbs (parsley, cilantro) in a handful

For the Vinaigrette:

- One tablespoon of olive oil
- One tablespoon of lemon juice
- One teaspoon Dijon mustard
- To taste, add salt and pepper.

DIRECTIONS

1. The cooked quinoa, sliced chicken, diced veggies, and crumbled feta cheese (if using) should all be combined in a bowl.
2. For the vinaigrette, combine the olive oil, lemon juice, Dijon mustard, salt, and pepper in a different container.
3. Drizzle the salad with the vinaigrette and toss to coat.

Before serving, add a fresh herb garnish.

Nutritional Information:

400 calories
30g of protein
10g of fat
35g of carbohydrates
5g of fiber

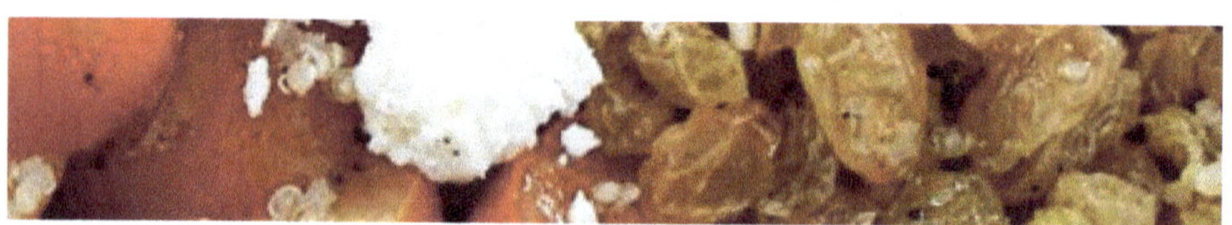

LENTIL SOUP WITH WHOLE-WHEAT BREAD

(Serves 1):

INGREDIENTS

- One cup of washed and drained canned lentils
- ½ cup chopped veggies (carrots, celery, onions) and one cup vegetable broth
- one minced garlic clove
- One teaspoon of dried thyme
- To taste, add salt and pepper.

One whole-wheat slice of bread

DIRECTIONS

1. Vegetable broth should be heated in a pot over medium heat. Vegetables should be chopped and cooked for 5 minutes to soften them.
2. Add the dried thyme, garlic, and lentils. Once the lentils are cooked, simmer for 20 to 25 minutes on low heat after bringing to a boil.
3. To taste, add salt and pepper for seasoning.

Serve warm, accompanied with a whole-wheat bread slice for dipping.

Nutritional Information:

350 calories

18g of protein

5g of fat

50g of carbohydrates

12g of fiber

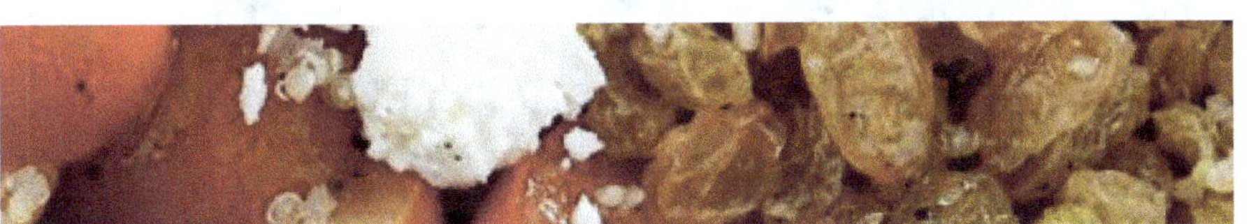

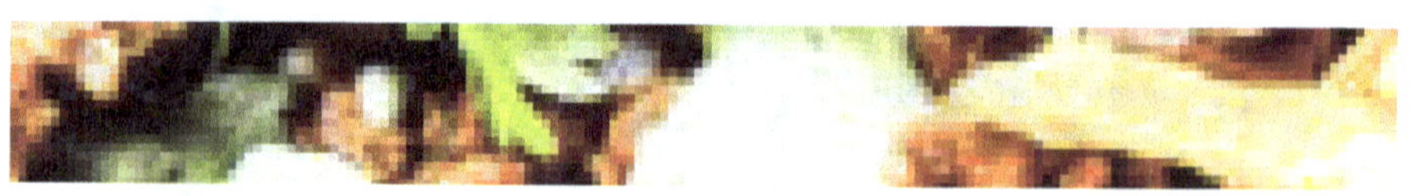

TURKEY TACO SALAD WITH COLORFUL VEGETABLES

(Serves 1):

INGREDIENTS

- Two ounces of cooked and seasoned ground turkey breast
- ½ cup of mixed greens
- ¼ cup finely chopped veggies, such as bell peppers, black beans, and corn
- Two tablespoons of salsa
- One tablespoon of shredded Monterey Jack or cheddar cheese

One tablespoon of diced avocado (optional)

DIRECTIONS

1. Mix the cooked ground turkey, chopped vegetables, shredded cheese, salsa, and avocado (if using) in a bowl.

Toss to coat, then relish!

Nutritional Information:
300 calories
Protein (25g) and Fat (10g)
20g of carbohydrates
5g of fiber

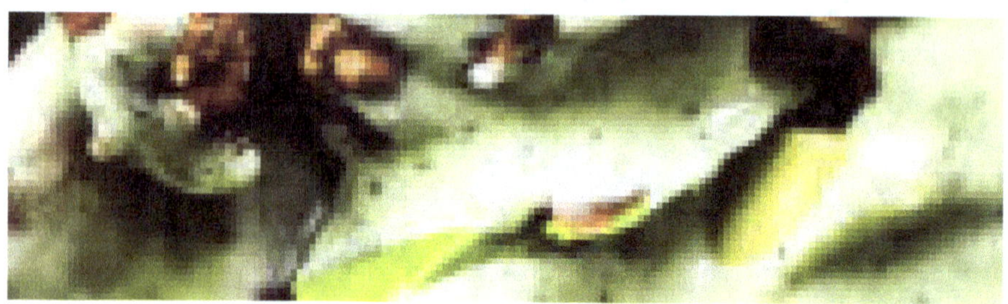

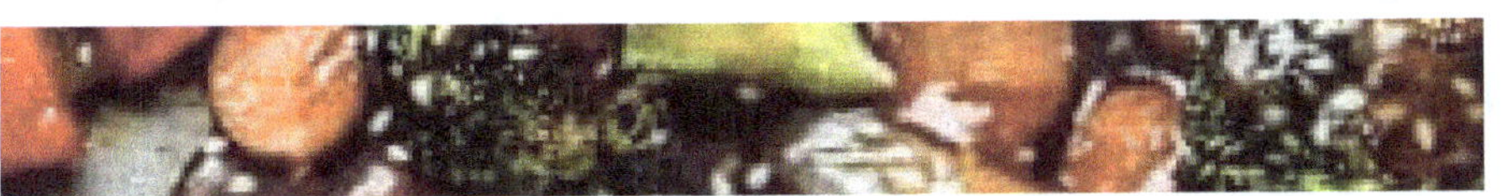

LEFTOVER SALMON WITH ROASTED VEGETABLES

(Serves 1):

INGREDIENTS

- 3 ounces of leftover baked or grilled salmon
- 1/4 cup of roasted veggies, such as Brussels sprouts, asparagus, and broccoli
- 1 tablespoon cooked whole-wheat couscous
- 1 tablespoon (optional) balsamic glaze

DIRECTIONS

1. Warm up any leftover salmon (cook using preferred technique if grilling or baking fresh).
2. Reheat the roasted veggies (if using fresh, preheat the oven to 400°F/200°C and bake for 15 to 20 minutes, or until they are soft).
3. In a bowl, mix cooked couscous, roasted veggies, and salmon.
- Enjoy after adding a balsamic glaze drizzle (optional).

Nutritional Information:

Note: Nutritional information will vary depending on the cooking method of the salmon and vegetables. (Example values based on grilled salmon and roasted broccoli):

Calories: 400

Protein: 35g

Fat: 15g

Carbs: 25g

Fiber: 5g

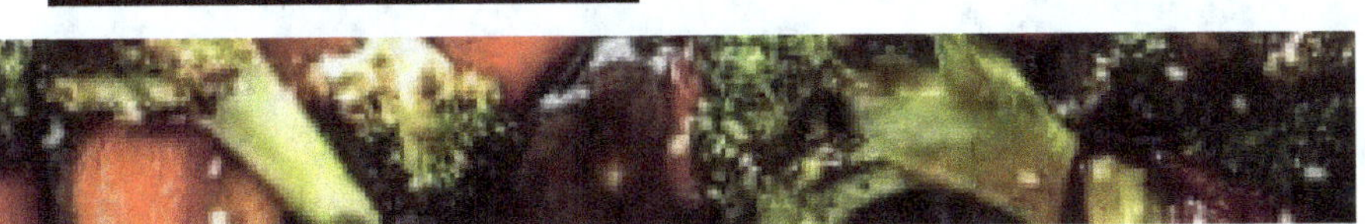

TUNA SALAD LETTUCE WRAPS

(Serves 1):

INGREDIENTS

- 2 ounces of flaked canned tuna in water and ¼ cup of chopped celery
- Chop 1 tablespoon of red onion
- One tablespoon of light mayo
- One teaspoon of lemon juice
- One-third teaspoon dried dill
- To taste, add salt and pepper.
- Two huge leaves of romaine lettuce

DIRECTIONS

1. Mix chopped celery, red onion, mayonnaise, lemon juice, dried dill, salt, and pepper with the flaked tuna in a bowl.
2. Lettuce romaine should be washed and dried.
3. Spoon combination of tuna salad onto middle of each lettuce leaf.
- To make a lettuce leaf wrap, fold the bottom up and roll it securely.

Nutritional Information:
250 calories
20g of protein, 10g of fat
5g of carbohydrates
2g of fiber

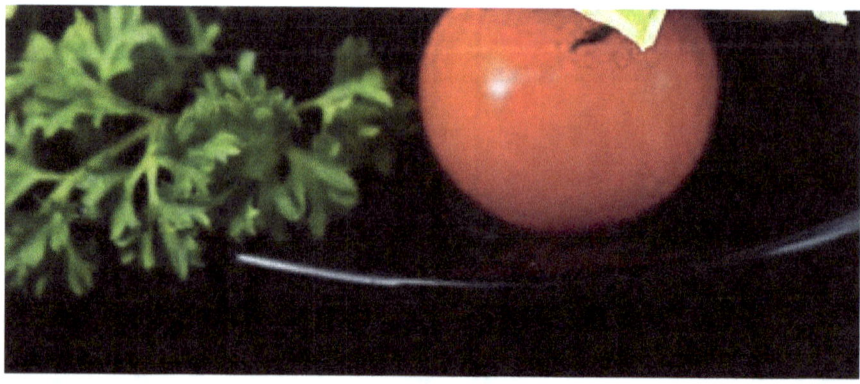

TUNA SALAD LETTUCE WRAPS

(Serves 1):

INGREDIENTS

- 2 ounces of flaked canned tuna in water and ¼ cup of chopped celery
- Chop 1 tablespoon of red onion
- One tablespoon of light mayo
- One teaspoon of lemon juice
- One-third teaspoon dried dill
- To taste, add salt and pepper.
- Two huge leaves of romaine lettuce

DIRECTIONS

1. Mix chopped celery, red onion, mayonnaise, lemon juice, dried dill, salt, and pepper with the flaked tuna in a bowl.
2. Lettuce romaine should be washed and dried.
3. Spoon combination of tuna salad onto middle of each lettuce leaf.
- To make a lettuce leaf wrap, fold the bottom up and roll it securely.

Nutritional Information:
250 calories
20g of protein, 10g of fat
5g of carbohydrates
2g of fiber

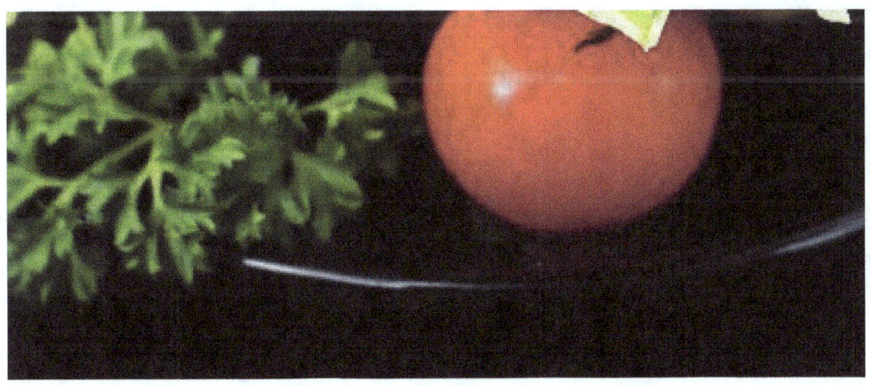

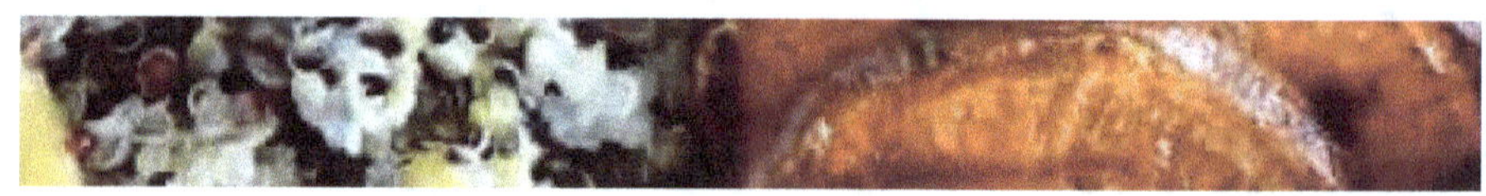

CHICKPEA VEGGIE BUDDHA BOWL

(Serves 1):

INGREDIENTS

- ½ cup of cooked, drained and rinsed chickpeas
- ½ cup finely chopped veggies (cucumbers, carrots, broccoli)
- 1/4 cup of cooked quinoa
- Optional: 2 tablespoons of crumbled feta cheese
- One tablespoon of hummus
- 1 tablespoon freshly chopped parsley

DIRECTIONS

1. Put cooked chickpeas, chopped veggies, cooked quinoa, feta cheese crumbles (if using), hummus, and chopped parsley in a bowl.
2. Toss to coat, then relish!

Nutritional Information:
350 calories
15g of protein
15g of fat
35g of carbohydrates
8g of fiber

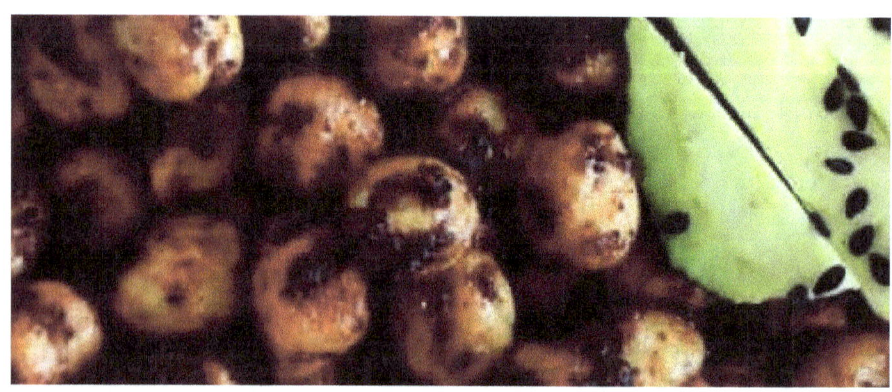

CREAMY TOMATO SOUP WITH WHOLE-WHEAT TOAST (Serves 1):

INGREDIENTS

- One cup of undrained canned diced tomatoes
- 1/4 cup vegetable broth and ½ cup of finely chopped veggies (onions, carrots)
- One tablespoon light cream cheese
- One teaspoon of dried basil
- To taste, add salt and pepper.
- One slice of whole-wheat bread

DIRECTIONS

1. Diced tomatoes, chopped veggies, vegetable broth, and dried basil should all be combined in a saucepan.
2. When the vegetables are tender, reduce the heat and simmer for 15 minutes after bringing to a boil.
3. Take off the stove and blend in the light cream cheese until it melts and becomes creamy.
4. To taste, add salt and pepper for seasoning.
5. Serve warm, accompanied by a whole-wheat bread slice for dipping.

Nutritional Information:

250 calories

10g of protein

5g of fat

35g of carbohydrates

5g of fiber

CHICKEN CAESAR SALAD WITH LIGHT DRESSING (Serves 1):

INGREDIENTS

- Slicing 3 ounces of grilled chicken breast and 2 cups of mixed greens
- Half a cup of cherry tomatoes
- One tablespoon grated Parmesan cheese
- Half a tablespoon of light Caesar dressing

DIRECTIONS

1. Add sliced chicken breast, cherry tomatoes, grated Parmesan cheese, and mixed greens to a bowl.
2. Toss to coat, then drizzle with a light Caesar salad dressing.

Nutritional Information:

350 calories

30g of protein

10g of fat

15g of carbohydrates

2g of fiber

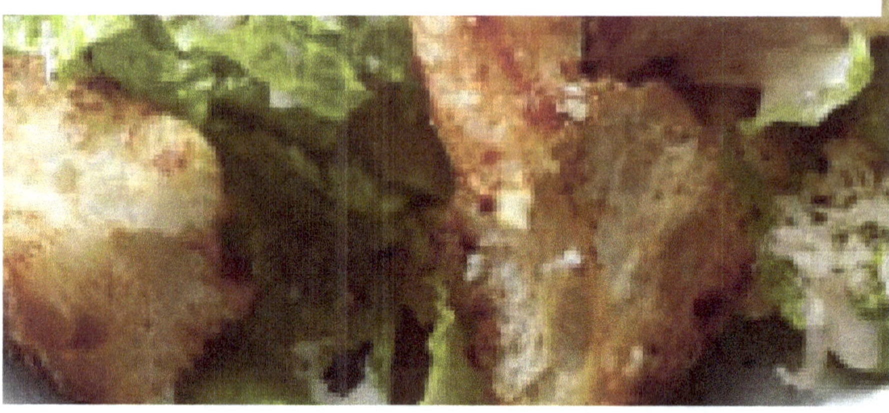

TURKEY AND VEGGIE PITA POCKETS

(Serves 1):

INGREDIENTS

- One warmed whole-wheat pita bread
- Two-ounce slices of turkey breast
- ¼ cup of finely cut veggies, such as bell peppers, cucumbers, and lettuce
- One tablespoon of hummus
- 1 tablespoon of feta cheese crumbles (optional)

DIRECTIONS

1. Eat a whole-wheat pita bread warm, as directed on the package.
2. Spread the pita bread with hummus inside.
3. Add the chopped veggies, sliced turkey breast, and crumbled feta cheese (if using).
4. The pita bread should be folded with the sides and bottom facing the center, then folded in half to form a pocket.

Nutritional Information:

300 calories

25g of protein

10g of fat

30g of carbohydrates

5g of fiber

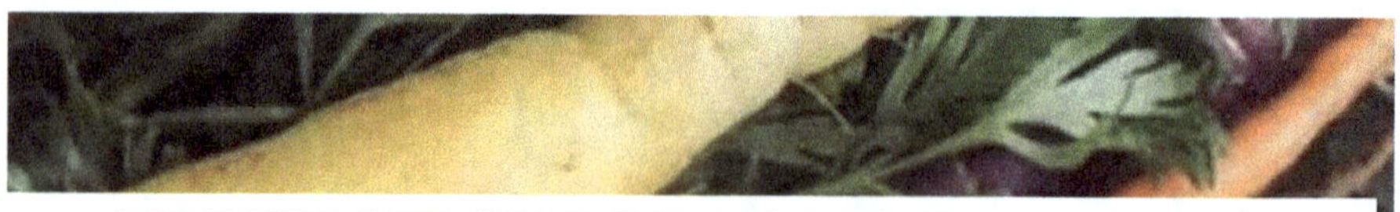

EDAMAME SNACK BOX WITH CARROT STICKS AND HUMMUS   (Serves 1):

INGREDIENTS

- ½ cup cooked and cooled shelled edamame
- ½ cup baby carrots
- Two tablespoons of hummus

DIRECTIONS

1. Baby carrots and cooked, chilled edamame should be combined in a container.
2. Add hummus to a different container so that you can dip it in.

Nutritional Information:

200 calories

12g of protein

5g of fat

20g of carbohydrates

8g of fiber

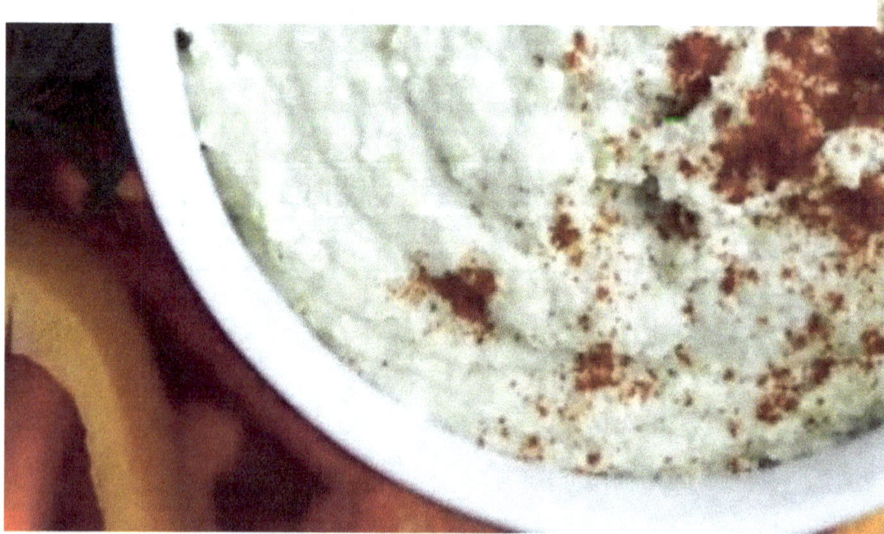

You can keep your afternoons full of energy and your metabolism boosted with these ten tasty and simple lunch ideas. You may break free from the dreary lunch routine and discover a world of delectable possibilities that will fuel your hectic day with these portable and gourmet options!

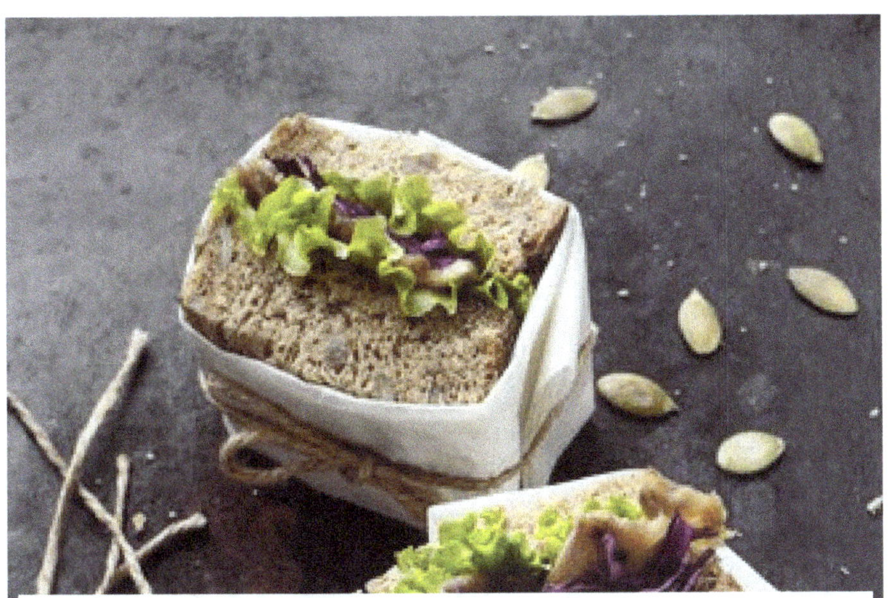

PART 2: DINNERTIME DELIGHTS - NOURISHING MEALS FOR A REVVING METABOLISM

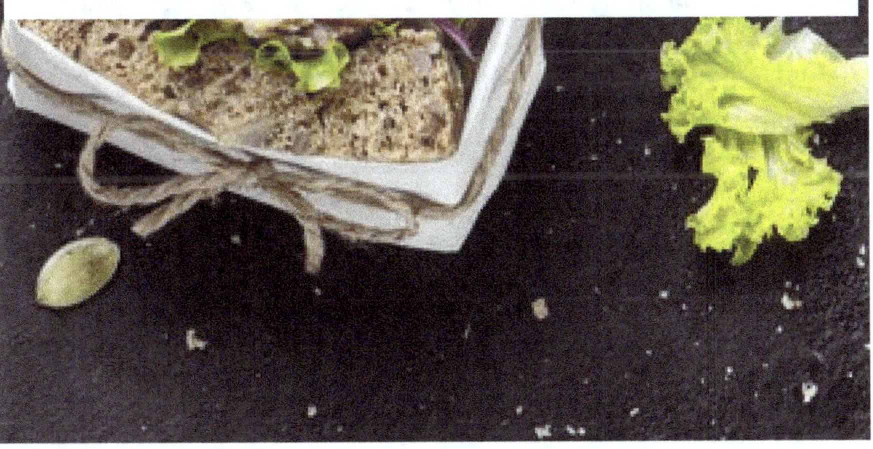

WEEKNIGHT WONDERS - SIMPLE & SPEEDY DINNERS FOR WOMEN ON THE GO

Dinner dash is a true challenge! Who has time for fancy meals with work, errands, and family obligations? Busy woman, do not fear! This chapter is a treasure trove of quick, easy, and nutritious meal recipes.

We will look at some recipes that are:

Quick & Simple: After a demanding day, there's no need to rush to the takeout menu. Even the busiest schedules can accommodate these dinners, which may be prepared in 30 minutes or less.

Delicious & Filling: Not everything that is quick has to be boring! These meals are full of flavor that will nourish your body and please your palate.

Minimal Cleanup: After a hard day, we realize you don't want to spend hours cleaning. These meals are made to be easily cleaned up after, which reduces stress after supper.

Prepare to explore a world of tasty supper options that are **quick, flavorful, and fuss-free** by throwing away the takeout routine. Together, let's cook delicious meals—even on the busiest weeknights!

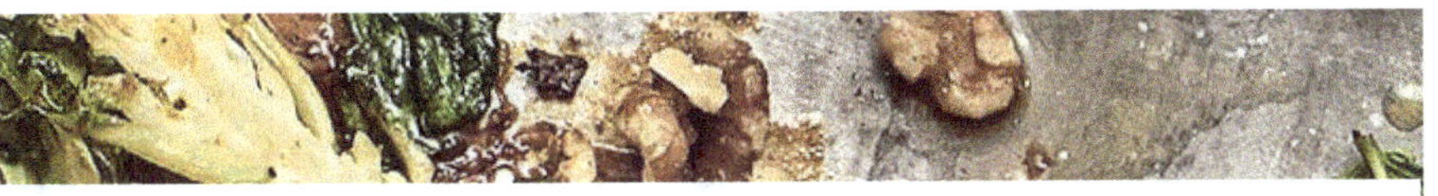

ONE-PAN SALMON WITH ROASTED BRUSSELS SPROUTS AND QUINOA (Serves 2):

INGREDIENTS

- Two 4-ounce salmon fillets apiece
- Half a cup of cleaned and trimmed Brussels sprouts
- 1/4 cup of washed quinoa
- One tablespoon of olive oil
- One teaspoon of dried thyme
- Half a cup of vegetable stock
- To taste, add salt and pepper.

DIRECTIONS

1. Turn the oven on to 400°F, or 200°C.
2. On a baking sheet, toss Brussels sprouts with olive oil, thyme, salt, and pepper.
3. After rinsing, distribute the quinoa in a single layer around the baking sheet's Brussels sprouts.
4. Top the quinoa and veggies with the salmon fillets.
5. Fill the baking sheet's bottom with vegetable broth.
6. Bake for 20 to 25 minutes, or until the veggies are soft and the salmon is cooked through.

Nutritional Information (per serving)

450 calories

30g of protein

20g of fat

35g of carbohydrates

5g of fiber

SLOW COOKER VEGETARIAN CHILI WITH KIDNEY BEANS, BLACK BEANS, AND CORN

(Serves 4):

INGREDIENTS

- One can (15 oz) of chopped, undrained tomatoes
- One can (15 oz) of washed and drained kidney beans
- One can (15 oz) of rinsed and drained black beans
- one cup of corn, frozen
- ½ cup finely chopped onion
- One sliced green bell pepper
- two minced garlic cloves
- One teaspoon of chili powder
- One teaspoon of cumin
- One-half teaspoon of dried oregano
- Four cups of broth made with vegetables

DIRECTIONS

1. Put all ingredients into a slow cooker and stir.
2. Once the chili is well-heated and thickened, simmer it on low for 6–8 hours or on high for 4–5 hours, stirring frequently.

Nutritional Information (per serving)

300 calories
Protein (15g) and Fat (5g)
45g of carbohydrates
10g of fiber

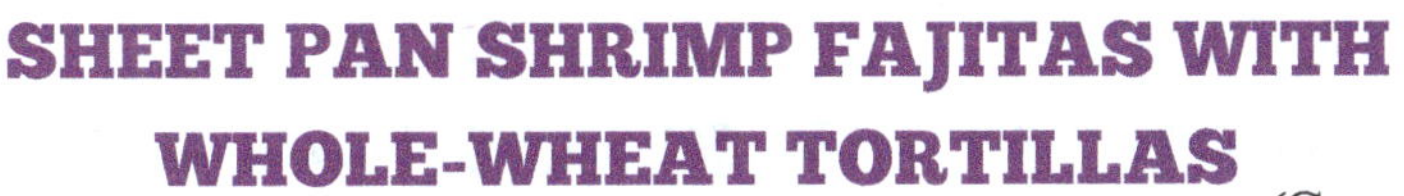

SHEET PAN SHRIMP FAJITAS WITH WHOLE-WHEAT TORTILLAS

(Serves 2):

INGREDIENTS

- 12 ounces of peeled and deveined shrimp
- One sliced bell pepper and one sliced red onion
- One tablespoon of olive oil
- One teaspoon of chili powder
- One-half teaspoon cumin
- 1/4 teaspoon smoked paprika
- To taste, add salt and pepper.
- Two tacos made using whole wheat
- Extra toppings at your discretion: salsa, diced avocado, and reduced-fat Greek yogurt

DIRECTIONS

1. Turn the oven on to 400°F, or 200°C.
2. Add olive oil, smoked paprika, cumin, chili powder, and pepper to the shrimp, bell peppers, and onion.
3. Arrange the mixture in a single layer on a baking sheet.
4. Bake for 15 to 20 minutes, or until the vegetables are crisp-tender and the shrimp are cooked through.
5. Reheat whole-wheat tortillas as directed on the package.
6. Top the shrimp fajita mixture with selected toppings and serve with warmed tortillas.

Nutritional Information
(per serving)

400 calories
Protein (35g) and Fat (15g)
30g of carbohydrates
2g of fiber

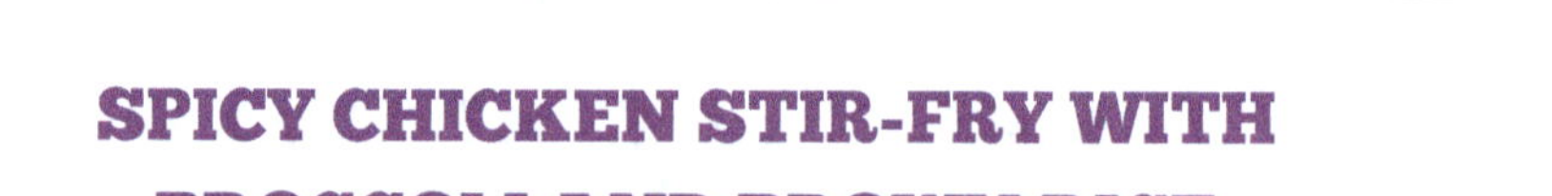

SPICY CHICKEN STIR-FRY WITH BROCCOLI AND BROWN RICE   (Serves 2):

INGREDIENTS

- Two skinless, boneless chicken breasts, thinly sliced
- one cup florets of broccoli
- ½ cup of brown rice, cooked
- One tablespoon of soy sauce
- One tablespoon of rice vinegar
- One teaspoon Sriracha (modify for desired amount of spiciness)
- One teaspoon cornstarch
- Spoonful of vegetable oil
- one minced garlic clove
- 1 tsp finely chopped ginger, optional
- To taste, add salt and pepper.

DIRECTIONS

1. Combine the cornstarch, sriracha, rice vinegar, and soy sauce in a small bowl. Put aside.
2. In a large skillet or wok, heat the vegetable oil over medium-high heat. Cook the chicken for five to seven minutes, or until it is thoroughly cooked and browned.
3. If using, add the ginger and garlic, and simmer, stirring constantly, for 30 seconds.
4. Cook the broccoli florets for a further two to three minutes, or until they are crisp-tender.
5. After adding the soy sauce mixture to the pan, simmer it. Simmer the sauce for one minute, or until it slightly thickens.
6. Add the cooked brown rice and fully heat it.
7. To taste, add salt and pepper for seasoning.

TURKEY BURGERS WITH SWEET POTATO FRIES

(Serves 2):

INGREDIENTS

For the Turkey Burgers:

- One pound of turkey breast meat
- A quarter of a cup finely chopped red bell pepper and onion
- Half a cup of panko breadcrumbs
- One tablespoon Worcestershire sauce
- One teaspoon of dried thyme
- To taste, add salt and pepper.

For the Sweet Potato Fries:

- wedges sliced from one medium sweet potato
- One tablespoon of olive oil
- 1/2 tsp paprika 1/2 tsp garlic powder
- To taste, add salt and pepper.

DIRECTIONS

1. Turn the oven on to 400°F, or 200°C.
2. Ground turkey, onion, bell pepper, panko breadcrumbs, Worcestershire sauce, thyme, salt, and pepper should all be combined in a big basin. Toss to blend well.
3. Divide the batter into two equal portions.
4. Sweet potato wedges should be tossed with olive oil, salt, pepper, paprika, and garlic powder. Arrange in a single layer on a baking sheet.
5. In a skillet, preheat to medium. When the turkey burgers are heated through, add them and cook for four to five minutes on each side.
6. Sweet potato wedges should be baked for 20 to 25 minutes, or until they are crisp-tender, turning them over halfway through.
7. Present sweet potato fries alongside turkey burgers.

CREAMY TOMATO PASTA WITH SPINACH AND CHICKEN SAUSAGE

(Serves 2):

INGREDIENTS

- 8 ounces of whole-wheat pasta
- 1 cup of fresh or canned chopped tomatoes
- ½ cup ricotta cheese, reduced fat
- Half a cup of finely chopped spinach
- 4 ounces of cooked and sliced chicken sausage
- One tablespoon of olive oil
- one minced garlic clove
- One-half teaspoon of dried oregano
- To taste, add salt and pepper.

DIRECTIONS

1. Follow the directions on the package to cook whole-wheat pasta.
2. Heat the olive oil in a big skillet over medium heat while the pasta cooks. Stir continuously for 30 seconds after adding the garlic.
3. Add the oregano and chopped tomatoes. Simmer until the tomatoes are tender, about 5 minutes.
4. Add spinach and ricotta cheese and stir. Cook until spinach is wilted, about 1 more minute.
5. To taste, add salt and pepper for seasoning.
6. After draining, combine the cooked pasta with the sliced chicken sausage and tomato sauce mixture.

Nutritional Information (per serving)

450 calories
30g of protein
15g of fat
45g of carbohydrates
5g of fiber

ONE-PAN LEMON GARLIC SALMON WITH ROASTED ASPARAGUS (Serves 2):

INGREDIENTS

- Two 4-ounce salmon fillets apiece
- One cut bunch of asparagus
- One tablespoon of olive oil
- One tablespoon of lemon juice
- One teaspoon of garlic powder
- Half a teaspoon of dried thyme
- To taste, add salt and pepper.

DIRECTIONS

1. Turn the oven on to 400°F, or 200°C.
2. Add garlic powder, thyme, olive oil, lemon juice, salt, and pepper to the asparagus and toss.
3. Place the asparagus on a baking sheet in a single layer.
4. Arrange the salmon fillets over the asparagus.
5. Bake for 15 to 20 minutes, or until the asparagus is crisp-tender and the salmon is cooked through.

Nutritional Information (per serving)

400 calories
35g protein and 20g fat.
15g of carbohydrates
2g of fiber

CHICKEN AND VEGETABLE STIR-FRY WITH BROWN RICE NOODLES (Serves 2):

INGREDIENTS

- Two skinless, boneless chicken breasts, thinly sliced
- One cup of mixed veggies, such as carrots, snap peas, and broccoli florets
- Cooked brown rice noodles, ½ cup
- One tablespoon of soy sauce
- One tablespoon of rice vinegar
- One teaspoon of sesame oil
- One teaspoon cornstarch
- Spoonful of vegetable oil
- one minced garlic clove
- 1 tsp finely chopped ginger, optional
- To taste, add salt and pepper.

DIRECTIONS

1. Mix the cornstarch, sesame oil, rice vinegar, and soy sauce in a small basin. Put aside.
2. In a large skillet or wok, heat the vegetable oil over medium-high heat. Cook the chicken for five to seven minutes, or until it is thoroughly cooked and browned.
3. If using, add the ginger and garlic, and simmer, stirring constantly, for 30 seconds.
4. When the vegetables are crisp-tender, add the mixed veggies and simmer for a further two to three minutes.
5. After adding the soy sauce mixture to the pan, simmer it. Simmer the sauce for one minute, or until it slightly thickens.
6. Add the cooked brown rice noodles and fully cook them.
7. To taste, add salt and pepper for seasoning.

Nutritional Information (per serving):

450 calories

30g of protein

15g of fat

40g of carbohydrates

5g of fiber

LENTIL SOUP WITH WHOLE-WHEAT BREAD AND A SIDE SALAD (Serves 2):

INGREDIENTS

- One cup of rinsed and sorted dried lentils
- One cup of chopped veggies (carrots, celery, onions) and four cups of vegetable broth
- one minced garlic clove
- One teaspoon of dried thyme

To taste, add salt and pepper.

For the Side Salad:

- Various greens
- One tablespoon of olive oil
- One tablespoon of lemon juice

To taste, add salt and pepper.

DIRECTIONS

1. Lentils, chopped veggies, vegetable broth, garlic, and thyme should all be combined in a big saucepan.
2. After bringing to a boil, lower the heat, and simmer the lentils for 30 to 35 minutes, or until they become soft.
3. To taste, add salt and pepper for seasoning.

For the Side Salad:

1. Combine mixed greens, lemon juice, olive oil, salt, and pepper in a bowl.

Nutritional Information (per serving):

400 calories

18g of protein, 5g of fat

60g of carbohydrates

15g of fiber

These ten quick and simple dinner recipes are a tasty and nourishing approach to maintain a high metabolism all week long. You may prepare filling meals that easily fit into your hectic schedule with little preparation or cleanup. Have fun!

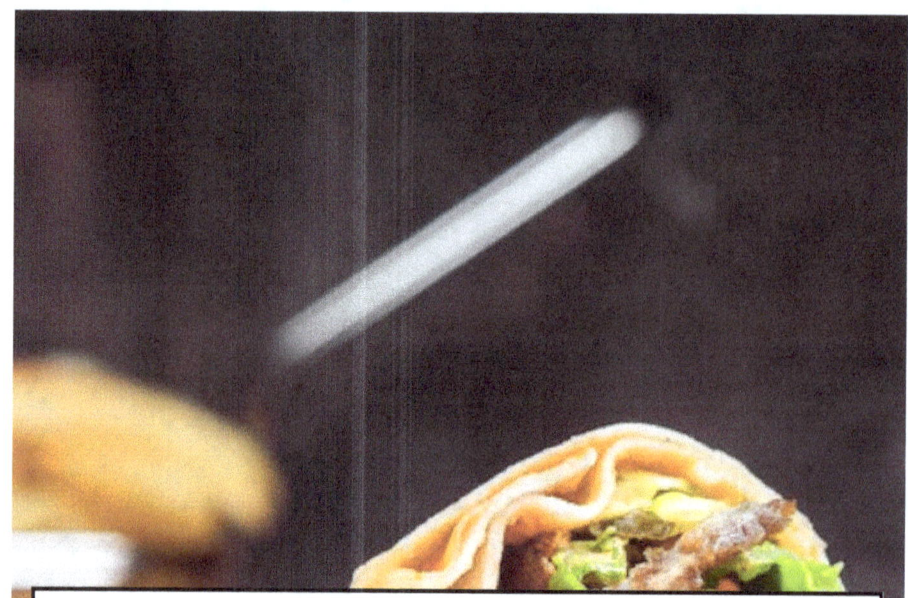

PART 3: SNACK SAVVY - SMART BITES FOR SUSTAINED ENERGY

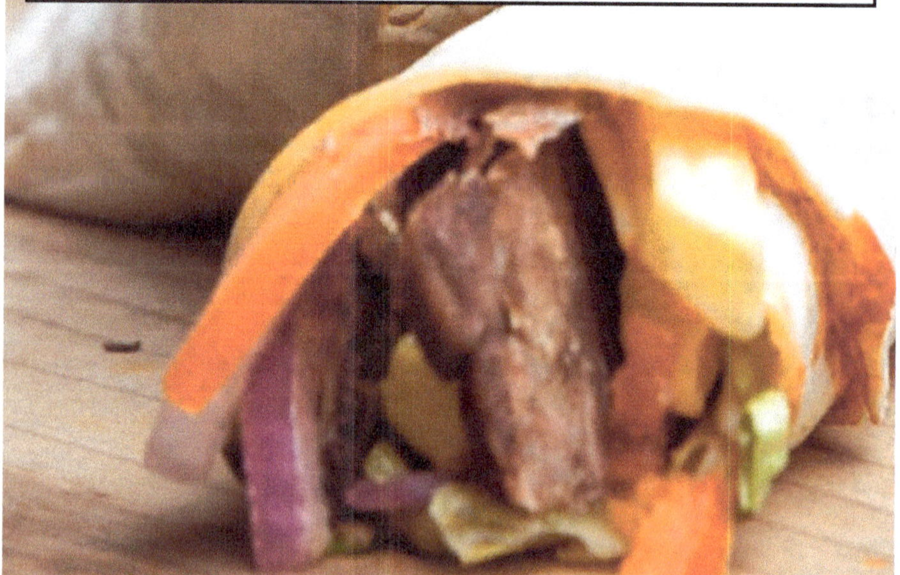

BEYOND THE BAG - DITCH THE PROCESSED & CRAFT HEALTHY SNACKS

Feeling peckish in between meals? Go beyond the cookie or chip bag! This chapter gives you the information and ideas you need to make **scrumptious and healthy homemade snacks.**

We'll look at a range of choices, including:

Easy & Content: This is not a place for intricate recipes! You can quickly prepare these snacks to keep yourself full and energized all day.

Perfect & Transportable: Your healthy decisions shouldn't be undermined by hectic schedules. These portable snacks are perfect for keeping you energized no matter where life takes you.

Delectable: Give up the extra sugars and artificial flavors. These snacks will keep your taste buds satisfied and your body nourished because they are packed with of natural sweetness and fresh ingredients.

Prepare to explore a world of scrumptious and healthful homemade snack alternatives by throwing out your commercial munchies! Together, let's set out on this delicious adventure!

PROTEIN POWER BITES

(Makes about 12 bites)

INGREDIENTS

- half a cup of rolled oats
- ¼ cup of unsweetened cashew, peanut, or almond butter
- half a cup of dried fruit (chopped cranberries, raisins, and dates)
- half a cup of chia seeds

two tsp honey

DIRECTIONS

1. Mix all the ingredients together in a big bowl.
2. Scoop the mixture onto a baking sheet covered with parchment paper, making bite-sized portions with a spoon.
3. To give them time to set, refrigerate for a minimum of thirty minutes.

**Nutritional Information
(per bite, approx.)**

100 calories
4g of protein
5g of fat
12g of carbohydrates
2g of fiber

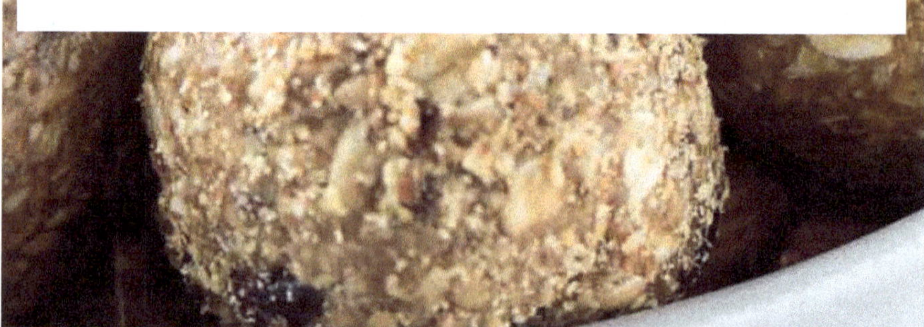

EDAMAME WITH SPICY GARLIC DIP

(Serves 1):

INGREDIENTS

- One cup of frozen peas, thawed ¼ cup of low-fat Greek yogurt
- one minced garlic clove
- A pinch of optional red pepper flakes

To taste, add salt and pepper.

DIRECTIONS

1. Follow the directions on the package to cook the edamame. After draining, rinse under cold water.
2. Greek yogurt, garlic, red pepper flakes (if using), salt, and pepper should all be combined in a small bowl.
3. Put the yogurt dip on the side for dipping the edamame.

**Nutritional Information
(per bite, approx.)**

150 calories
12g of protein
5g of fat
10g of carbohydrates
5g of fiber

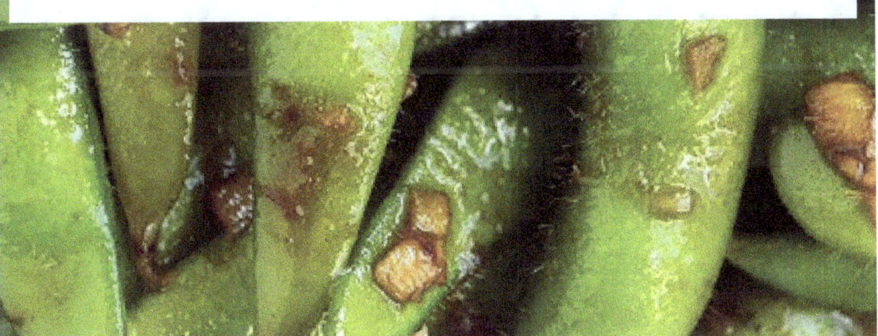

YOGURT PARFAIT WITH BERRIES AND GRANOLA (Serves 1):

INGREDIENTS

- ½ cup of Greek yogurt, plain
- ½ cup of fresh berries, such as raspberries, strawberries, and blueberries
- ¼ cup of granola (choose low-sugar or unsweetened varieties)
- One tablespoon of almonds, slivered (optional)

DIRECTIONS

1. Arrange a quarter cup of Greek yogurt and a quarter cup of fruit in a little container or parfait glass.
2. Once more, arrange the yogurt and berries in layers.
3. Sprinkle granola and, if desired, slivered almonds on top.

Nutritional Information (per bite, approx.)

300 calories
Protein (15g) and Fat (10g)
30g of carbohydrates
5g of fiber

COTTAGE CHEESE WITH PINEAPPLE AND CHIA SEEDS (Serves 1):

INGREDIENTS

- ½ cup cottage cheese with little fat
- ¼ cup of freshly cut pineapple
- One spoonful of chia seeds
- Honey drizzle (optional)

DIRECTIONS

1. Place the cottage cheese, chia seeds, and diced pineapple in a bowl.
2. If desired, drizzle with honey to add a little sweetness.

Nutritional Information
(per bite, approx.)

150 calories

18g of protein

3g of fat

15g of carbohydrates

2g of fiber

APPLE SLICES WITH ALMOND BUTTER

(Serves 1):

INGREDIENTS

- One sliced apple and two teaspoons of almond butter

DIRECTIONS

1. Slice and clean your apple.
2. Toast apple slices and spread with almond butter for dipping.

Nutritional Information
(per bite, approx.)

200 calories
4g of protein
8g of fat
25g of carbohydrates
4g of fiber

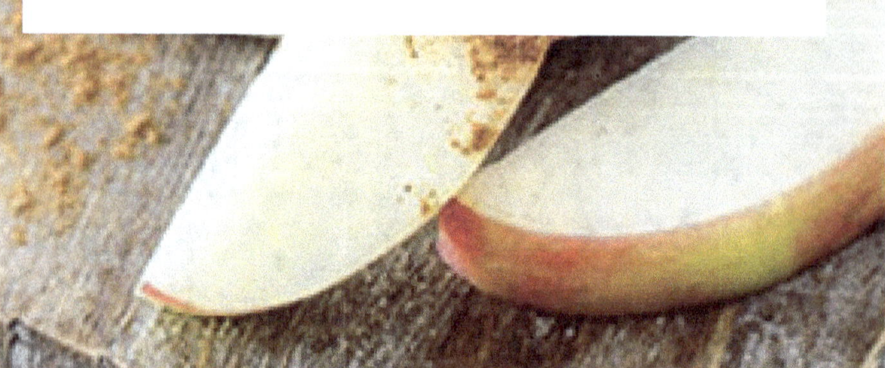

BELL PEPPER SLICES WITH HUMMUS

(Serves 1)

INGREDIENTS

- One bell pepper, cut into thin strips
- ½ cup hummus (choose a flavor you like)

DIRECTIONS

1. Peel and cut the bell pepper into long, thin strips.
2. Present bell pepper slices beside hummus for dunks.

Nutritional Information
(per bite, approx.)

200 calories

5g of protein

8g of fat

20g of carbohydrates

3g of fiber

TRAIL MIX WITH NUTS, SEEDS, AND DRIED FRUIT (Makes about 1 cup)

INGREDIENTS

- Half a cup of uncooked almonds
- ¼ cup of cranberries, dried
- Half a cup of pumpkin seeds
- ¼ cup finely chopped dried apricots (or any other preferred dried fruit)
- Additions that are optional: Dark chocolate chips with shredded coconut (use sparingly)

DIRECTIONS

1. Mix all ingredients together in a bowl.
2. Keep in an airtight container for convenient on-the-go access.

Nutritional Information (per ¼ cup serving, approx.):

200 calories

5g protein and 10g fat.

20g of carbohydrates

3g of fiber

COTTAGE CHEESE WITH CUCUMBER AND DILL   (Serves 1)

INGREDIENTS

- Half a cup of uncooked almonds
- ¼ cup of cranberries, dried
- Half a cup of pumpkin seeds
- ¼ cup finely chopped dried apricots (or any other preferred dried fruit)
- Additions that are optional: Dark chocolate chips with shredded coconut (use sparingly)

DIRECTIONS

1. Mix all ingredients together in a bowl.
2. Keep in an airtight container for convenient on-the-go access.

Nutritional Information (per ¼ cup serving, approx.):

200 calories

5g protein and 10g fat.

20g of carbohydrates

3g of fiber

GREEK YOGURT WITH BERRIES AND FLAXSEED (Serves 1)

INGREDIENTS

- ½ cup of Greek yogurt, plain
- ½ cup of fresh berries, such as raspberries, strawberries, and blueberries
- One spoonful of flaxseed meal

DIRECTIONS

1. Fresh berries and Greek yogurt should be combined in a bowl.
2. Top with a dusting of ground flaxseed.

Nutritional Information (per ¼ cup serving, approx.):

200 calories
Protein (15g) and Fat (5g)
20g of carbohydrates
4g of fiber

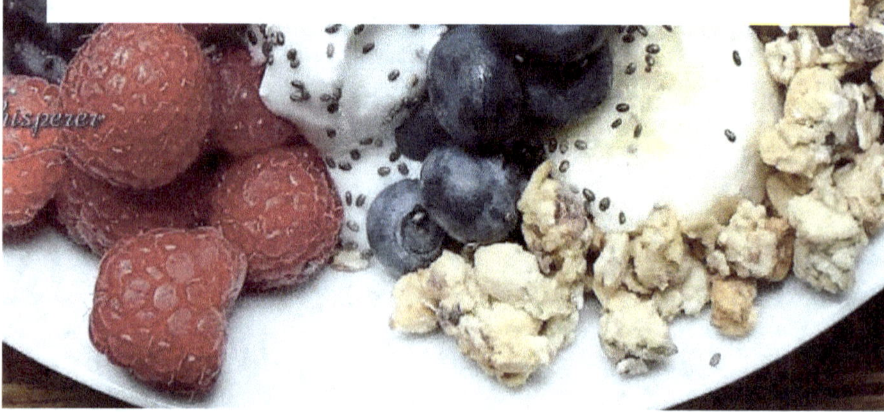

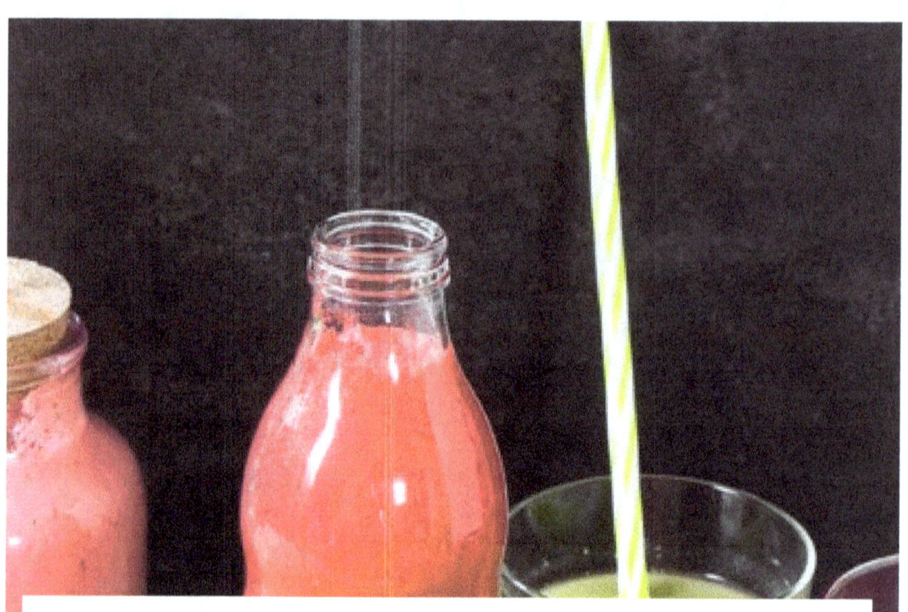

SMOOTHIES FOR METABOLISM

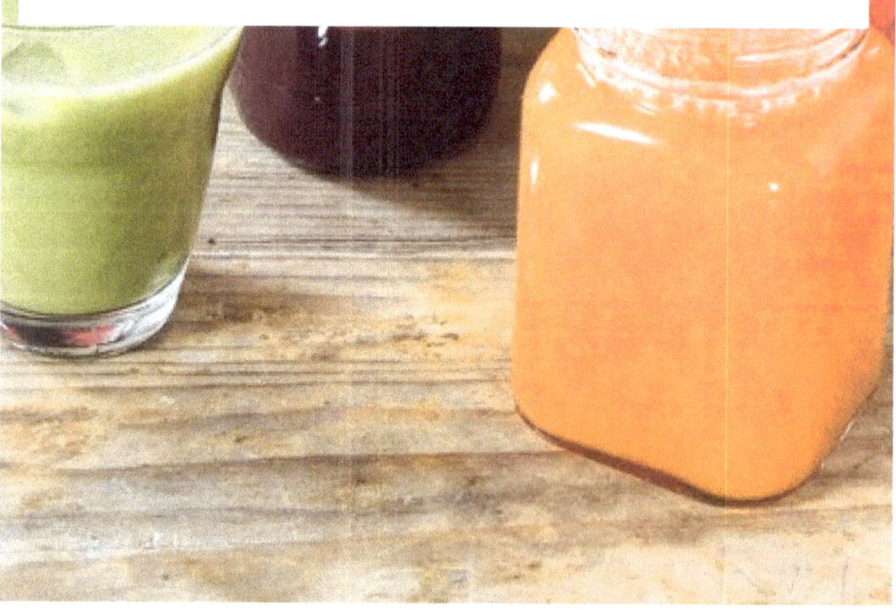

GREEN TEA GINGER BLAST

(Serves 1)

INGREDIENTS

- One cup of chilled brewed green tea
- Half a banana
- One knob of chopped, peeled ginger
- One scoop of vanilla or unflavored protein powder
- ½ cup spinach

DIRECTIONS

1. Blend each item until it becomes creamy and smooth.

Nutritional Information (approx.):

250 calories

Protein (20g) and Fat (5g)

20g of carbohydrates

4g of fiber

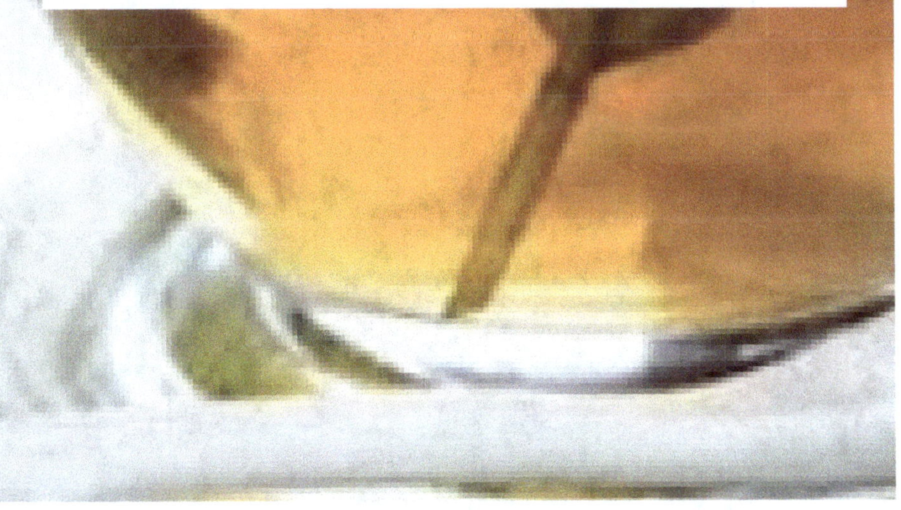

BERRY PROTEIN POWER

(Serves 1)

INGREDIENTS

- 1 cup of mixed berries, either frozen or fresh
- ½ cup of Greek yogurt, plain
- Half a cup of almond milk
- One spoonful of chia seeds
- A handful of baby spinach

DIRECTIONS

1. Blend each item until it becomes creamy and smooth.

Nutritional Information (approx.):

300 calories
Protein (20g) and Fat (5g)
30g of carbohydrates
6g of fiber

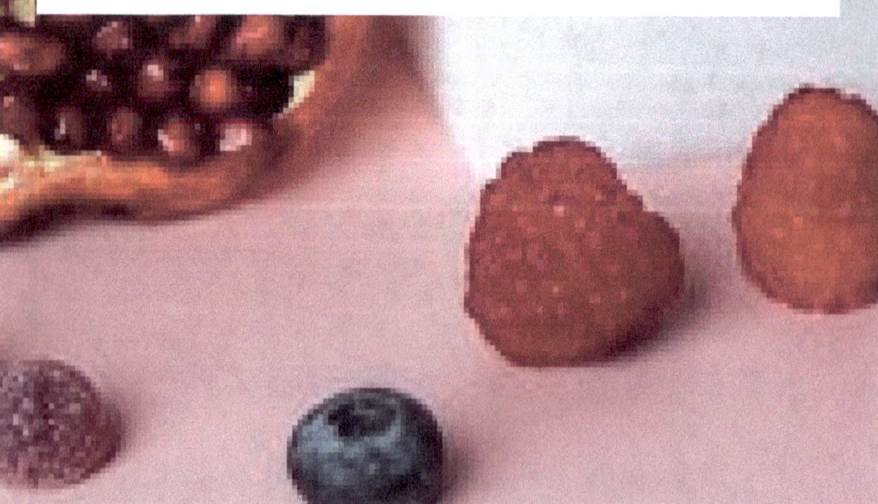

TROPICAL FAT BURNER

(Serves 1)

INGREDIENTS

- One cup of chopped pineapple, fresh or frozen
- ½ cup mango chunks, either fresh or frozen
- One cup of sugar-free coconut water
- Just a small bunch of kale leaves
- Squeeze lime juice

DIRECTIONS

1. Blend each item until it becomes creamy and smooth.

Nutritional Information (approx.):

200 calories
Meat: 2g, Fat: 1g
45g of carbohydrates
3g of fiber

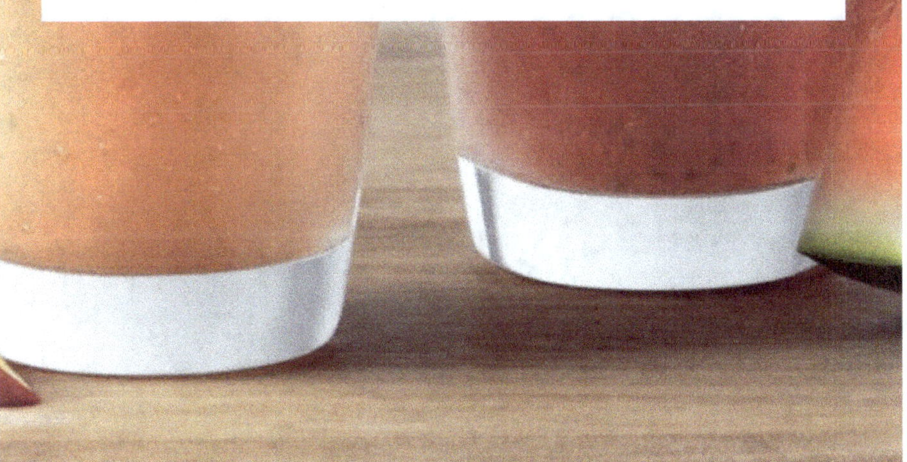

CREAMY COFFEE KICK

(Serves 1)

INGREDIENTS

- One cup of cooled brewed coffee
- ½ cup of Greek yogurt, plain
- Half a banana
- One spoonful of butter made of almonds
- One-half teaspoon of ground cinnamon

DIRECTIONS

1. Blend each item until it becomes creamy and smooth.

Nutritional Information (approx.):

300 calories
Protein (15g) and Fat (10g)
25g of carbohydrates
2g of fiber

GREEN GLOW SMOOTHIE

(Serves 1)

INGREDIENTS

- one cup of spinach
- Half a banana
- ½ cup pieces of frozen mango
- one cup of water
- One tablespoon of optional chia seeds

DIRECTIONS

1. Blend each item until it becomes creamy and smooth.

Nutritional Information (approx.):

200 calories

2g of protein

Fat: 1 gram

40g of carbohydrates

5g of fiber (chia seeds included)

BEET IT UP SMOOTHIE

(Serves 1)

INGREDIENTS

- One cup of cooked beets (frozen or fresh)
- Half a banana
- ½ cup of Greek yogurt, plain
- 1/4 cup carrot juice
- Half a cup water
- A pinch of ginger powder

DIRECTIONS

1. Blend each item until it becomes creamy and smooth.

Nutritional Information (approx.):

250 calories

10g of protein

5g of fat

30g of carbohydrates

3g of fiber

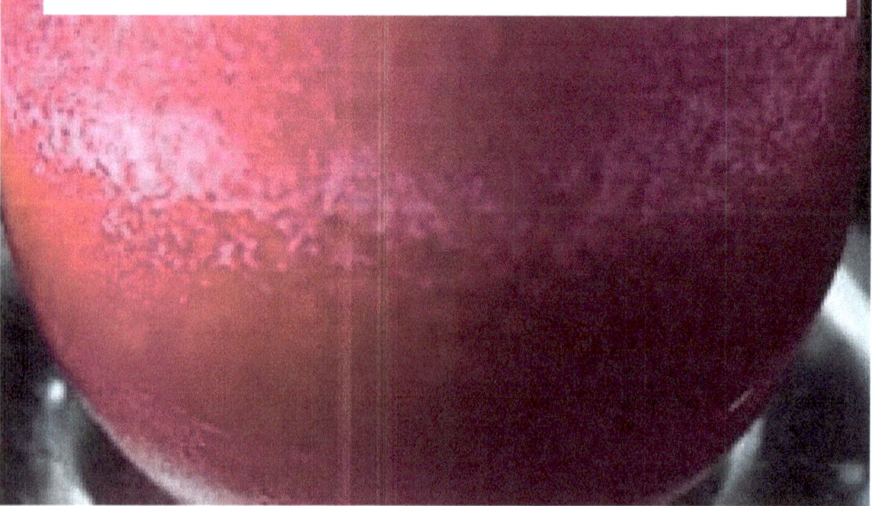

CITRUS SUNSHINE SMOOTHIE

(Serves 1)

INGREDIENTS

- One peeled grapefruit or ½ cup of grapefruit juice
- One peeled orange, or ½ cup of orange juice
- Half a banana
- One cup of finely chopped kale
- Half a cup of water

DIRECTIONS

1. Blend each item until it becomes creamy and smooth.

Nutritional Information (approx.):

200 calories

3g of protein

Fat: 1 gram

45g of carbohydrates

4g of fiber

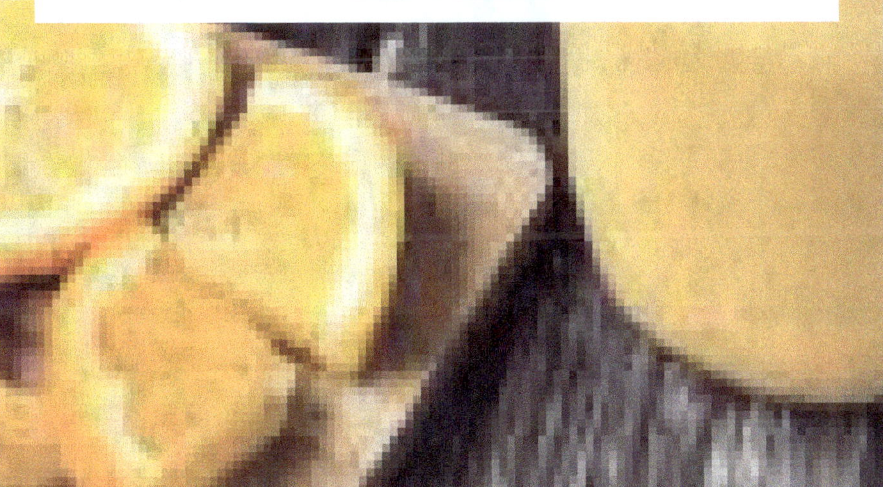

MATCHA GREEN GOODNESS

(Serves 1)

INGREDIENTS

- 1 cup almond milk without sugar
- Half a banana
- One scoop of matcha powder
- One handful of baby spinach
- One spoonful of honey, if desired

DIRECTIONS

1. Blend each item until it becomes creamy and smooth.

Nutritional Information (approx.):

200 calories

4g of protein

5g of fat

25g of carbohydrates

2g of fiber

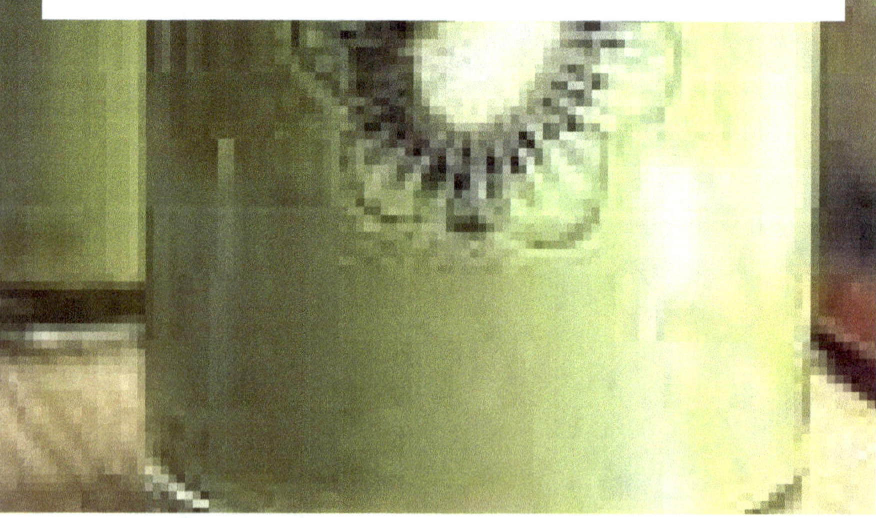

CHOCOLATE CHERRY RECOVERY

(Serves 1)

INGREDIENTS

- 1 cup unsweetened tart cherry juice
- Half a banana
- Half a cup of frozen cherries
- One scoop of protein powder with chocolate flavor
- A handful of baby spinach

DIRECTIONS

1. Blend each item until it becomes creamy and smooth.

Nutritional Information (approx.):

250 calories

Protein (20g) and Fat (5g)

25g of carbohydrates

3g of fiber

SPICE UP YOUR LIFE - CULINARY HERBS & SPICES THAT BOOST YOUR METABOLISM

Are you looking for a healthy approach to boost your **metabolism and add flavor and fire to your meals?** You only need to look to the colorful world of spices and herbs! This chapter delves further into the fascinating world of these influential chefs.

We'll look at a range of spices and herbs that have benefits beyond flavor. You'll learn how these components can:

Boost Your Metabolism Naturally: Your body may burn calories more effectively by using certain herbs and spices, which will assist your metabolism.

Add Flavor Without Adding Sugar or Sodium: Replace your unhealthy seasonings with tasty substitutes to give your food a boost of flavor.

Boost General Health: A variety of herbs and spices are rich in components that are good for you overall, including antioxidants.

Prepare to discover a wealth of taste and usefulness! Join us as we investigate how adding herbs and spices to your meals might change them and possibly even speed up your metabolism.

THE POWER OF PLANTS: EXPLORING SPICES WITH METABOLIC BENEFITS

Spices have been used for purposes other than flavoring food for ages. Their capacity to preserve food and their medical qualities made them highly valued. However, did you know that some spices may also have an unexpectedly positive effect on your metabolism?

Our bodies are intricate machinery, and the process by which we turn food into energy is called metabolism. We can keep a healthy weight and energy level by maintaining a healthy metabolism. Exercise and diet are important factors, but adding some spices can help naturally.

The following are some common spices that may improve your metabolism:

1. Chili Peppers: The chemical capsaicin, which gives chili peppers their fiery kick, may enhance thermogenesis, the body's process of producing heat. There may be a little increase in calories burned as a result.

2. Ginger: Known for its digestive properties, this adaptable root may also have an impact on metabolism. According to studies, ginger may aid with insulin sensitivity and blood sugar regulation, two things that affect metabolism.

3. Turmeric: The plant's primary ingredient, curcumin, has strong anti-inflammatory and possibly metabolic properties.

Curcumin may help control cholesterol, blood sugar, and possibly even enhance calorie burning, according to research.

4. Cinnamon: You may get sweetness without adding more sugar by using this warming spice. Additionally, cinnamon may aid in blood sugar regulation, which may tangentially aid in metabolism. Research indicates that it may enhance insulin sensitivity, enabling your body to utilize glucose more efficiently.

5. Black pepper: A common kitchen ingredient, black pepper may have a thermogenic impact akin to that of chili peppers in addition to enhancing flavors. The main ingredient in black pepper, piperine, may speed up metabolism and improve nutritional absorption.

MAXIMIZING THE POWER OF SPICES:

The best results from spices come from regular use in a balanced diet and way of life. To get the most out of them, consider these suggestions:

- **Variety Is Essential:** Don't restrict yourself to one or two types of spices. Try out various combinations to produce intriguing flavor profiles and possibly gain additional metabolic advantages.
- **Best Fresh:** Although dried spices are more handy, fresh herbs and spices have the potential to have higher quantities of therapeutic components and a more intense flavor.

- **Match with Nutritious Foods:** Spices can enhance the flavor of nutritious foods, which can motivate you to choose them more frequently.

EXPLORING THE WORLD OF SPICES:

You may add a little magic to your food and possibly give your body a natural boost by adding these and other metabolism-boosting spices to your meals. So embrace your inner chef, learn about the fascinating world of spices, and set out on a tasty path to better health!

RECIPES HIGHLIGHTING METABOLISM-BOOSTING SPICES

Spicy Scrambled Eggs with Turmeric and Black Pepper: For a breakfast high in protein and boosting the metabolism, scramble eggs with chopped veggies (tomatoes, spinach), turmeric powder, black pepper, and (optional) chili flakes.

Greek Yogurt with Berries and Cinnamon: To make a sweet and filling breakfast that may help control blood sugar levels, mix plain Greek yogurt with fresh berries, ground cinnamon, and honey.

Green Power Smoothie with Ginger: Blend spinach, banana, frozen mango, water, and a small amount of grated ginger to make a revitalizing and metabolism-boosting smoothie. In addition to perhaps enhancing insulin sensitivity, ginger may help with digestion.

SWEET DREAMS FOR A REVVED METABOLISM - SLEEP & THE POWER OF RECOVERY

Ever wonder why sleeping well feels so rejuvenating? It goes beyond simply feeling refreshed! Your overall health, especially your metabolism, is greatly impacted by getting enough sleep. We explore the intriguing relationship between sleep and metabolism in this chapter.

We'll look at how sleep is:

Effects on Hormone Regulation: Your body releases hormones that control hunger and metabolism when you sleep. This delicate balance can be upset by getting too little sleep, which may result in increased appetites and a slow metabolism.

Encourages Muscle Recovery: Your body rebuilds and repairs muscle tissue as you sleep. Since muscle consumes more calories at rest than fat tissue, this mechanism is necessary to keep the metabolism in a healthy range.

Reduces Stress: Your metabolism might suffer greatly from long-term stress. Sleep gives your body the much-needed respite from the grind of daily life that it needs to regulate stress hormones and maybe maintain a balanced metabolic rate.

Prepare to unleash the potential of sleep to boost your metabolism! This chapter will help you improve your evening routine and establish healthy sleep habits so that you wake up feeling better and more invigorated. So put on your best pajamas, turn down the lights, and get ready to learn how having beautiful dreams can help you become a more metabolically efficient version of yourself!

THE SCIENCE OF SLEEP & METABOLISM: WHY REST MATTERS

Many people value sleep highly and frequently forgo it in the rush of everyday life. Beyond the obvious effects of weariness and drowsiness, however, sleeping too little can seriously affect your metabolism—the mechanism by which your body turns food into energy. Knowing the science underlying the relationship between metabolism and sleep might serve as a strong incentive to prioritize those valuable evening hours.

The Hormonal Orchestra of Sleep and Metabolism:

Hormones interact delicately to control many intricate processes within our body. In this metabolic orchestra, leptin and ghrelin are two important instruments. Ghrelin, which is produced in the stomach, increases hunger, but leptin, which is produced by fat cells, indicates satiety (feeling full).

Leptin levels rise and ghrelin levels fall when we sleep. This hormonal harmony helps to maintain a healthy calorie balance by encouraging feelings of fullness and discouraging overeating. Sleep deprivation, however, upsets this equilibrium. Research has indicated that insufficient sleep might result in a reduction in leptin synthesis and an increase in ghrelin synthesis, which may heighten cravings and excessive eating.

Sleep and Muscle Repair: The Metabolic Engine

The function of muscle tissue in metabolism is vital. greater muscle mass results in a greater metabolic rate because muscles burn more calories at rest than fat tissue. Muscle tissue is strained during waking hours by our regular activities. Sleep offers a crucial opportunity for reconstruction and healing.

Human growth hormone (HGH), which encourages muscle growth and repair, is released by the body during deep sleep. Getting enough sleep guarantees that HGH is produced at the best possible level, which helps with muscle recovery and maintains a healthy metabolic rate.

The Stress Connection: How Sleep Impacts Metabolism

Chronic stress is a modern epidemic, and it has detrimental implications that go well beyond mental health. Stress chemicals such as cortisol have the ability to interfere with several body processes, including metabolism. Stress raises cortisol levels in the body, which may increase blood sugar and cause fat to be stored.

The body can properly regulate stress hormones when it gets enough sleep. We improve the conditions for a healthy metabolism when we sleep by letting cortisol levels return to normal.

The Bottom Line: Prioritizing Sleep for a Revved Metabolism

The science is in: your metabolism may suffer if you don't get enough sleep. Lack of sleep can cause weight gain and make it harder to maintain a healthy weight by upsetting hormonal balance, impeding muscle regeneration, and raising stress hormones.

- It's important to aim for 7-8 hours of good sleep per night for the best metabolic performance. Here are some pointers to encourage sound sleeping practices:

- Create a regular sleep routine by going to bed and waking up at the same times every day, even on the weekends.

- Establish a calming nighttime routine: Before going to bed, unwind with peaceful pursuits like reading or having a warm bath.

- Improve the conditions under which you sleep by keeping your bedroom cold, quiet, and dark.

- Reduce the amount of time you spend using screens before bed because the blue light they emit can interfere with your sleep.

- Steer clear of alcohol and caffeine right before bed: These drugs may affect how well you sleep.

You're supporting your metabolism, enhancing general health and well-being, and investing in your energy and mood when you prioritize sleep and develop appropriate sleep habits. Give your metabolism the gift of a restful night's sleep by turning out the lights and going to bed!

CREATING A SLEEP SANCTUARY: TIPS FOR A GOOD NIGHT'S REST

Getting a decent night's sleep can seem like a luxury in the fast-paced world of today. Apart from the instant advantages of feeling rejuvenated and invigorated, getting enough sleep is essential for preserving a robust immune system, a balanced metabolism, and general wellbeing. This chapter explores the art of setting up a sleep sanctuary, a haven created especially to encourage sound sleep and enhance your evening ritual.

The Power of Environment:

Our sleeping environment has a significant effect on the quality of our sleep. We may greatly increase our chances of waking up feeling rested and revitalized by setting up an environment that encourages calm and deep sleep.

Light it Up (or Down):

Light is a potent modulator of our circadian rhythm. The hormone melatonin, which indicates tiredness, can be suppressed by exposure to intense light, particularly in the evening. Here's how to maximize the amount of light in your sleeping area:

- **Reduce the amount of light pollution:** Use eye masks or blackout drapes to block out external light sources.
- **Dim the lights:** In the evening, stay away from bright overhead lighting. Choose lamps with warmer, gentler tones to create a calm atmosphere.
- **Accept natural light:** When the day comes, pull back your curtains and let the light stream into the space. By regulating your circadian rhythm, this aids in maintaining a normal sleep-wake cycle.

Setting the Stage for Serenity:

Another significant sleep-disturbing factor is noise. Here are some pointers for setting up a calm and quiet sleeping space:

- **Purchase a white noise machine or earplugs:** While a white noise machine can produce a masking sound to assist drown out distracting stimuli, earplugs can be used to block out unpleasant sounds.
- **Reduce external noise:** If you live in a noisy neighborhood, you might want to think about soundproofing your doors or windows.

Temperature Matters:

As our bodies get ready for sleep, they naturally cool down. This process can be hampered by an uncomfortable bedroom, making it harder to fall or stay asleep.

- **Aim for a chilly temperature:** 60–67°F (15–19°C) is usually the best range for sleeping.
- Make an investment in breathable bedding by selecting blankets and sheets composed of natural fibers, such as cotton or linen, which promote better temperature control and ventilation.

Creating a Calming Atmosphere:

Rather of serving as a place to work or store things, your bedroom ought to be a peaceful retreat. Here are some ideas for establishing a soothing environment:

- **Clear the area:** It might be difficult to relax in a cluttered bedroom since it can be visually intimidating and uncomfortable. Make room for what you need and establish some order.
- **Relaxing Aromas:** Aromas with relaxing qualities include lavender, chamomile, and valerian root. To create a calming ambiance, think about using scented candles or essential oil diffusers (with discretion).
- **Calm Colors:** Use soothing paint hues for your bedroom walls, such as lavender, green, or blue. Stay away from vivid or energizing colors that can keep you up at night.

- Invest in Cozy Mattresses: A comfy mattress, plush pillows, and sheets are necessary for restful sleep.

The Power of Routine:

Routine is essential to our bodies, and sleep is no different. Your body's natural sleep-wake cycle can be regulated by creating a regular sleep routine, which can facilitate falling asleep and waking up feeling rested.

- Even on the weekends, go to bed and wake up at the same time every day.
- Establish a calming nighttime routine: Before going to bed, unwind with soothing pursuits like gentle stretching, a warm bath, or reading.
- Before going to bed, avoid engaging in stimulating activities: Try to avoid using screens (computers, phones, and TVs) for at least an hour before bed. Electronic gadget blue light has the potential to disrupt sleep.
- Create a bedtime routine that includes activities like reading a book, having a warm bath, or listening to relaxing music. Repetition assists your body in recognizing that It's time to relax and get ready for bed.

Beyond the Bedroom:

Although the atmosphere in your bedroom is very important for the quality of your sleep, good sleep practices don't end in your bedroom.

- Invest in Cozy Mattresses: A comfy mattress, plush pillows, and sheets are necessary for restful sleep.

The Power of Routine:

Routine is essential to our bodies, and sleep is no different. Your body's natural sleep-wake cycle can be regulated by creating a regular sleep routine, which can facilitate falling asleep and waking up feeling rested.

- Even on the weekends, go to bed and wake up at the same time every day.
- Establish a calming nighttime routine: Before going to bed, unwind with soothing pursuits like gentle stretching, a warm bath, or reading.
- Before going to bed, avoid engaging in stimulating activities: Try to avoid using screens (computers, phones, and TVs) for at least an hour before bed. Electronic gadget blue light has the potential to disrupt sleep.
- Create a bedtime routine that includes activities like reading a book, having a warm bath, or listening to relaxing music. Repetition assists your body in recognizing that It's time to relax and get ready for bed.

Beyond the Bedroom:

Although the atmosphere in your bedroom is very important for the quality of your sleep, good sleep practices don't end in your bedroom.

- **Frequent exercise:** Physical activity on a regular basis might enhance the quality of your sleep; however, avoid doing intense exercise right before bed.
- **Diet:** Your food and beverages have an effect on how well you sleep. Steer clear of alcohol, caffeine, and large meals right before bed.
- **Control your tension:** Prolonged stress might interfere with sleep. To reduce stress, engage in relaxation exercises like yoga, meditation, or deep breathing.
-

More than just a room's décor, a sleep sanctuary must be designed to complement your body's normal sleep-wake cycle and encourage restorative sleep. By using these suggestions and prioritizing your sleep, you can turn your bedroom into a peaceful retreat and harness the benefits of a restful night's sleep for a more vibrant, healthy you.

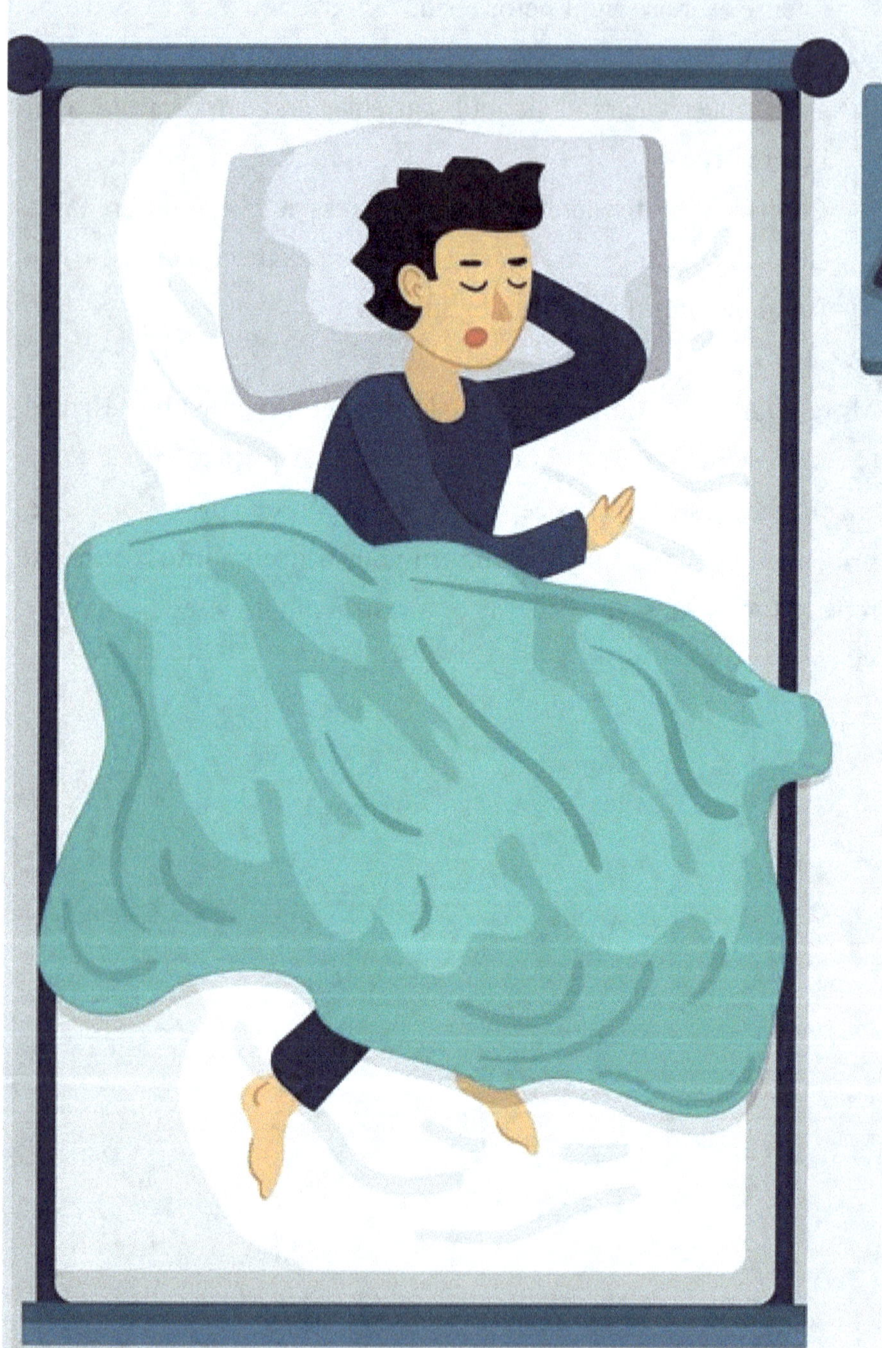

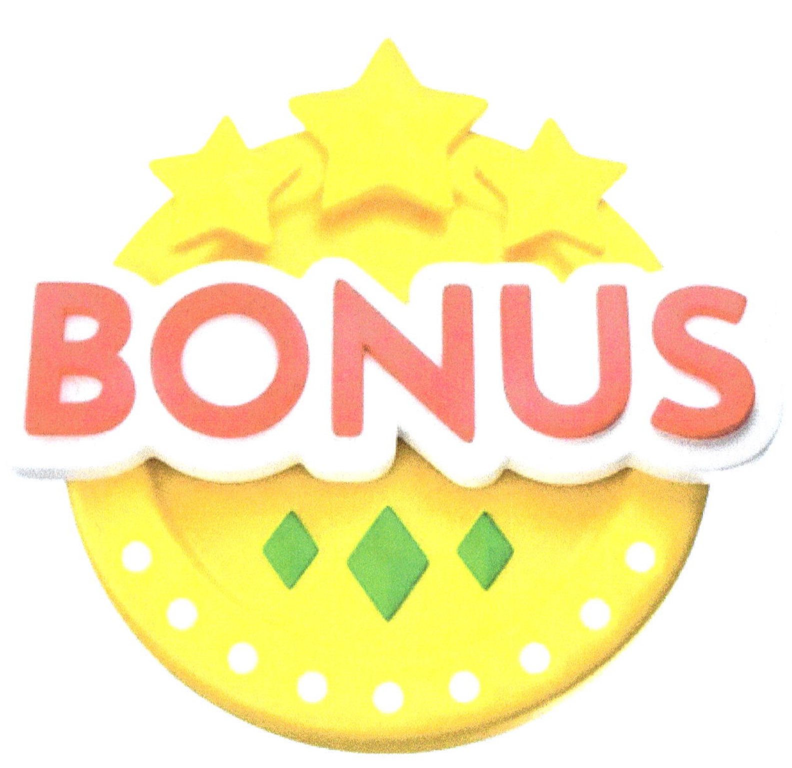
BONUS

WEEKLY MEAL PLANNER

MONDAY

BREAKFAST ___________________

LUNCH ___________________

SNACKS ___________________

DINNER ___________________

TUESDAY

BREAKFAST ___________________

LUNCH ___________________

SNACKS ___________________

DINNER ___________________

WEDNESDAY

BREAKFAST ___________________

LUNCH ___________________

SNACKS ___________________

DINNER ___________________

THURSDAY

BREAKFAST ___________________

LUNCH ___________________

SNACKS ___________________

DINNER ___________________

FRIDAY

BREAKFAST ___________________

LUNCH ___________________

SNACKS ___________________

DINNER ___________________

SATURDAY

BREAKFAST ___________________

LUNCH ___________________

SNACKS ___________________

DINNER ___________________

SUNDAY

BREAKFAST ___________________

LUNCH ___________________

SNACKS ___________________

DINNER ___________________

NOTES

____

____

____

____

WEEKLY MEAL PLANNER

MONDAY

BREAKFAST ___________________

LUNCH ___________________

SNACKS ___________________

DINNER ___________________

TUESDAY

BREAKFAST ___________________

LUNCH ___________________

SNACKS ___________________

DINNER ___________________

WEDNESDAY

BREAKFAST ___________________

LUNCH ___________________

SNACKS ___________________

DINNER ___________________

THURSDAY

BREAKFAST ___________________

LUNCH ___________________

SNACKS ___________________

DINNER ___________________

FRIDAY

BREAKFAST ___________________

LUNCH ___________________

SNACKS ___________________

DINNER ___________________

SATURDAY

BREAKFAST ___________________

LUNCH ___________________

SNACKS ___________________

DINNER ___________________

SUNDAY

BREAKFAST ___________________

LUNCH ___________________

SNACKS ___________________

DINNER ___________________

NOTES

____

____

____

____

WEEKLY MEAL PLANNER

MONDAY

BREAKFAST _______________________

LUNCH _______________________

SNACKS _______________________

DINNER _______________________

TUESDAY

BREAKFAST _______________________

LUNCH _______________________

SNACKS _______________________

DINNER _______________________

WEDNESDAY

BREAKFAST _______________________

LUNCH _______________________

SNACKS _______________________

DINNER _______________________

THURSDAY

BREAKFAST _______________________

LUNCH _______________________

SNACKS _______________________

DINNER _______________________

FRIDAY

BREAKFAST _______________________

LUNCH _______________________

SNACKS _______________________

DINNER _______________________

SATURDAY

BREAKFAST _______________________

LUNCH _______________________

SNACKS _______________________

DINNER _______________________

SUNDAY

BREAKFAST _______________________

LUNCH _______________________

SNACKS _______________________

DINNER _______________________

NOTES

____

____

____

____

WEEKLY MEAL PLANNER

MONDAY

BREAKFAST _______________________

LUNCH _______________________

SNACKS _______________________

DINNER _______________________

TUESDAY

BREAKFAST _______________________

LUNCH _______________________

SNACKS _______________________

DINNER _______________________

WEDNESDAY

BREAKFAST _______________________

LUNCH _______________________

SNACKS _______________________

DINNER _______________________

THURSDAY

BREAKFAST _______________________

LUNCH _______________________

SNACKS _______________________

DINNER _______________________

FRIDAY

BREAKFAST _______________________

LUNCH _______________________

SNACKS _______________________

DINNER _______________________

SATURDAY

BREAKFAST _______________________

LUNCH _______________________

SNACKS _______________________

DINNER _______________________

SUNDAY

BREAKFAST _______________________

LUNCH _______________________

SNACKS _______________________

DINNER _______________________

NOTES

____

____

____

____

WEEKLY MEAL PLANNER

MONDAY

BREAKFAST _______________________

LUNCH _______________________

SNACKS _______________________

DINNER _______________________

TUESDAY

BREAKFAST _______________________

LUNCH _______________________

SNACKS _______________________

DINNER _______________________

WEDNESDAY

BREAKFAST _______________________

LUNCH _______________________

SNACKS _______________________

DINNER _______________________

THURSDAY

BREAKFAST _______________________

LUNCH _______________________

SNACKS _______________________

DINNER _______________________

FRIDAY

BREAKFAST _______________________

LUNCH _______________________

SNACKS _______________________

DINNER _______________________

SATURDAY

BREAKFAST _______________________

LUNCH _______________________

SNACKS _______________________

DINNER _______________________

SUNDAY

BREAKFAST _______________________

LUNCH _______________________

SNACKS _______________________

DINNER _______________________

NOTES

____

____

____

____

WEEKLY MEAL PLANNER

MONDAY

BREAKFAST _______________________

LUNCH _______________________

SNACKS _______________________

DINNER _______________________

TUESDAY

BREAKFAST _______________________

LUNCH _______________________

SNACKS _______________________

DINNER _______________________

WEDNESDAY

BREAKFAST _______________________

LUNCH _______________________

SNACKS _______________________

DINNER _______________________

THURSDAY

BREAKFAST _______________________

LUNCH _______________________

SNACKS _______________________

DINNER _______________________

FRIDAY

BREAKFAST _______________________

LUNCH _______________________

SNACKS _______________________

DINNER _______________________

SATURDAY

BREAKFAST _______________________

LUNCH _______________________

SNACKS _______________________

DINNER _______________________

SUNDAY

BREAKFAST _______________________

LUNCH _______________________

SNACKS _______________________

DINNER _______________________

NOTES

____

____

____

____

WEEKLY MEAL PLANNER

MONDAY
BREAKFAST ______________________
LUNCH ______________________
SNACKS ______________________
DINNER ______________________

TUESDAY
BREAKFAST ______________________
LUNCH ______________________
SNACKS ______________________
DINNER ______________________

WEDNESDAY
BREAKFAST ______________________
LUNCH ______________________
SNACKS ______________________
DINNER ______________________

THURSDAY
BREAKFAST ______________________
LUNCH ______________________
SNACKS ______________________
DINNER ______________________

FRIDAY
BREAKFAST ______________________
LUNCH ______________________
SNACKS ______________________
DINNER ______________________

SATURDAY
BREAKFAST ______________________
LUNCH ______________________
SNACKS ______________________
DINNER ______________________

SUNDAY
BREAKFAST ______________________
LUNCH ______________________
SNACKS ______________________
DINNER ______________________

NOTES
____
____
____
____

WEEKLY MEAL PLANNER

MONDAY

BREAKFAST _______________________

LUNCH _______________________

SNACKS _______________________

DINNER _______________________

TUESDAY

BREAKFAST _______________________

LUNCH _______________________

SNACKS _______________________

DINNER _______________________

WEDNESDAY

BREAKFAST _______________________

LUNCH _______________________

SNACKS _______________________

DINNER _______________________

THURSDAY

BREAKFAST _______________________

LUNCH _______________________

SNACKS _______________________

DINNER _______________________

FRIDAY

BREAKFAST _______________________

LUNCH _______________________

SNACKS _______________________

DINNER _______________________

SATURDAY

BREAKFAST _______________________

LUNCH _______________________

SNACKS _______________________

DINNER _______________________

SUNDAY

BREAKFAST _______________________

LUNCH _______________________

SNACKS _______________________

DINNER _______________________

NOTES

____

____

____

____

WEEKLY MEAL PLANNER

MONDAY

BREAKFAST _______________

LUNCH _______________

SNACKS _______________

DINNER _______________

TUESDAY

BREAKFAST _______________

LUNCH _______________

SNACKS _______________

DINNER _______________

WEDNESDAY

BREAKFAST _______________

LUNCH _______________

SNACKS _______________

DINNER _______________

THURSDAY

BREAKFAST _______________

LUNCH _______________

SNACKS _______________

DINNER _______________

FRIDAY

BREAKFAST _______________

LUNCH _______________

SNACKS _______________

DINNER _______________

SATURDAY

BREAKFAST _______________

LUNCH _______________

SNACKS _______________

DINNER _______________

SUNDAY

BREAKFAST _______________

LUNCH _______________

SNACKS _______________

DINNER _______________

NOTES

____

____

____

____

WEEKLY MEAL PLANNER

MONDAY

BREAKFAST __________________

LUNCH __________________

SNACKS __________________

DINNER __________________

TUESDAY

BREAKFAST __________________

LUNCH __________________

SNACKS __________________

DINNER __________________

WEDNESDAY

BREAKFAST __________________

LUNCH __________________

SNACKS __________________

DINNER __________________

THURSDAY

BREAKFAST __________________

LUNCH __________________

SNACKS __________________

DINNER __________________

FRIDAY

BREAKFAST __________________

LUNCH __________________

SNACKS __________________

DINNER __________________

SATURDAY

BREAKFAST __________________

LUNCH __________________

SNACKS __________________

DINNER __________________

SUNDAY

BREAKFAST __________________

LUNCH __________________

SNACKS __________________

DINNER __________________

NOTES

____

____

____

____

WEEKLY MEAL PLANNER

MONDAY

BREAKFAST _______________________

LUNCH _______________________

SNACKS _______________________

DINNER _______________________

TUESDAY

BREAKFAST _______________________

LUNCH _______________________

SNACKS _______________________

DINNER _______________________

WEDNESDAY

BREAKFAST _______________________

LUNCH _______________________

SNACKS _______________________

DINNER _______________________

THURSDAY

BREAKFAST _______________________

LUNCH _______________________

SNACKS _______________________

DINNER _______________________

FRIDAY

BREAKFAST _______________________

LUNCH _______________________

SNACKS _______________________

DINNER _______________________

SATURDAY

BREAKFAST _______________________

LUNCH _______________________

SNACKS _______________________

DINNER _______________________

SUNDAY

BREAKFAST _______________________

LUNCH _______________________

SNACKS _______________________

DINNER _______________________

NOTES

____

____

____

____

WEEKLY MEAL PLANNER

MONDAY

BREAKFAST _______________________

LUNCH _______________________

SNACKS _______________________

DINNER _______________________

TUESDAY

BREAKFAST _______________________

LUNCH _______________________

SNACKS _______________________

DINNER _______________________

WEDNESDAY

BREAKFAST _______________________

LUNCH _______________________

SNACKS _______________________

DINNER _______________________

THURSDAY

BREAKFAST _______________________

LUNCH _______________________

SNACKS _______________________

DINNER _______________________

FRIDAY

BREAKFAST _______________________

LUNCH _______________________

SNACKS _______________________

DINNER _______________________

SATURDAY

BREAKFAST _______________________

LUNCH _______________________

SNACKS _______________________

DINNER _______________________

SUNDAY

BREAKFAST _______________________

LUNCH _______________________

SNACKS _______________________

DINNER _______________________

NOTES

____

____

____

____

WEEKLY MEAL PLANNER

MONDAY

BREAKFAST ________________________

LUNCH ________________________

SNACKS ________________________

DINNER ________________________

TUESDAY

BREAKFAST ________________________

LUNCH ________________________

SNACKS ________________________

DINNER ________________________

WEDNESDAY

BREAKFAST ________________________

LUNCH ________________________

SNACKS ________________________

DINNER ________________________

THURSDAY

BREAKFAST ________________________

LUNCH ________________________

SNACKS ________________________

DINNER ________________________

FRIDAY

BREAKFAST ________________________

LUNCH ________________________

SNACKS ________________________

DINNER ________________________

SATURDAY

BREAKFAST ________________________

LUNCH ________________________

SNACKS ________________________

DINNER ________________________

SUNDAY

BREAKFAST ________________________

LUNCH ________________________

SNACKS ________________________

DINNER ________________________

NOTES

____

____

____

____

WEEKLY MEAL PLANNER

MONDAY

BREAKFAST _______________________

LUNCH _______________________

SNACKS _______________________

DINNER _______________________

TUESDAY

BREAKFAST _______________________

LUNCH _______________________

SNACKS _______________________

DINNER _______________________

WEDNESDAY

BREAKFAST _______________________

LUNCH _______________________

SNACKS _______________________

DINNER _______________________

THURSDAY

BREAKFAST _______________________

LUNCH _______________________

SNACKS _______________________

DINNER _______________________

FRIDAY

BREAKFAST _______________________

LUNCH _______________________

SNACKS _______________________

DINNER _______________________

SATURDAY

BREAKFAST _______________________

LUNCH _______________________

SNACKS _______________________

DINNER _______________________

SUNDAY

BREAKFAST _______________________

LUNCH _______________________

SNACKS _______________________

DINNER _______________________

NOTES

____

____

____

____

WEEKLY MEAL PLANNER

MONDAY

BREAKFAST ___________________

LUNCH ___________________

SNACKS ___________________

DINNER ___________________

TUESDAY

BREAKFAST ___________________

LUNCH ___________________

SNACKS ___________________

DINNER ___________________

WEDNESDAY

BREAKFAST ___________________

LUNCH ___________________

SNACKS ___________________

DINNER ___________________

THURSDAY

BREAKFAST ___________________

LUNCH ___________________

SNACKS ___________________

DINNER ___________________

FRIDAY

BREAKFAST ___________________

LUNCH ___________________

SNACKS ___________________

DINNER ___________________

SATURDAY

BREAKFAST ___________________

LUNCH ___________________

SNACKS ___________________

DINNER ___________________

SUNDAY

BREAKFAST ___________________

LUNCH ___________________

SNACKS ___________________

DINNER ___________________

NOTES

____

____

____

____

WEEKLY MEAL PLANNER

MONDAY

BREAKFAST _______________________

LUNCH _______________________

SNACKS _______________________

DINNER _______________________

TUESDAY

BREAKFAST _______________________

LUNCH _______________________

SNACKS _______________________

DINNER _______________________

WEDNESDAY

BREAKFAST _______________________

LUNCH _______________________

SNACKS _______________________

DINNER _______________________

THURSDAY

BREAKFAST _______________________

LUNCH _______________________

SNACKS _______________________

DINNER _______________________

FRIDAY

BREAKFAST _______________________

LUNCH _______________________

SNACKS _______________________

DINNER _______________________

SATURDAY

BREAKFAST _______________________

LUNCH _______________________

SNACKS _______________________

DINNER _______________________

SUNDAY

BREAKFAST _______________________

LUNCH _______________________

SNACKS _______________________

DINNER _______________________

NOTES

____

____

____

____

WEEKLY MEAL PLANNER

MONDAY

BREAKFAST _____________________

LUNCH _____________________

SNACKS _____________________

DINNER _____________________

TUESDAY

BREAKFAST _____________________

LUNCH _____________________

SNACKS _____________________

DINNER _____________________

WEDNESDAY

BREAKFAST _____________________

LUNCH _____________________

SNACKS _____________________

DINNER _____________________

THURSDAY

BREAKFAST _____________________

LUNCH _____________________

SNACKS _____________________

DINNER _____________________

FRIDAY

BREAKFAST _____________________

LUNCH _____________________

SNACKS _____________________

DINNER _____________________

SATURDAY

BREAKFAST _____________________

LUNCH _____________________

SNACKS _____________________

DINNER _____________________

SUNDAY

BREAKFAST _____________________

LUNCH _____________________

SNACKS _____________________

DINNER _____________________

NOTES

____

____

____

____

WEEKLY MEAL PLANNER

MONDAY

BREAKFAST _______________________

LUNCH _______________________

SNACKS _______________________

DINNER _______________________

TUESDAY

BREAKFAST _______________________

LUNCH _______________________

SNACKS _______________________

DINNER _______________________

WEDNESDAY

BREAKFAST _______________________

LUNCH _______________________

SNACKS _______________________

DINNER _______________________

THURSDAY

BREAKFAST _______________________

LUNCH _______________________

SNACKS _______________________

DINNER _______________________

FRIDAY

BREAKFAST _______________________

LUNCH _______________________

SNACKS _______________________

DINNER _______________________

SATURDAY

BREAKFAST _______________________

LUNCH _______________________

SNACKS _______________________

DINNER _______________________

SUNDAY

BREAKFAST _______________________

LUNCH _______________________

SNACKS _______________________

DINNER _______________________

NOTES

____

____

____

____

WEEKLY MEAL PLANNER

MONDAY

BREAKFAST _______________________

LUNCH _______________________

SNACKS _______________________

DINNER _______________________

TUESDAY

BREAKFAST _______________________

LUNCH _______________________

SNACKS _______________________

DINNER _______________________

WEDNESDAY

BREAKFAST _______________________

LUNCH _______________________

SNACKS _______________________

DINNER _______________________

THURSDAY

BREAKFAST _______________________

LUNCH _______________________

SNACKS _______________________

DINNER _______________________

FRIDAY

BREAKFAST _______________________

LUNCH _______________________

SNACKS _______________________

DINNER _______________________

SATURDAY

BREAKFAST _______________________

LUNCH _______________________

SNACKS _______________________

DINNER _______________________

SUNDAY

BREAKFAST _______________________

LUNCH _______________________

SNACKS _______________________

DINNER _______________________

NOTES

____

____

____

____

WEEKLY MEAL PLANNER

MONDAY

BREAKFAST _____________________

LUNCH _____________________

SNACKS _____________________

DINNER _____________________

TUESDAY

BREAKFAST _____________________

LUNCH _____________________

SNACKS _____________________

DINNER _____________________

WEDNESDAY

BREAKFAST _____________________

LUNCH _____________________

SNACKS _____________________

DINNER _____________________

THURSDAY

BREAKFAST _____________________

LUNCH _____________________

SNACKS _____________________

DINNER _____________________

FRIDAY

BREAKFAST _____________________

LUNCH _____________________

SNACKS _____________________

DINNER _____________________

SATURDAY

BREAKFAST _____________________

LUNCH _____________________

SNACKS _____________________

DINNER _____________________

SUNDAY

BREAKFAST _____________________

LUNCH _____________________

SNACKS _____________________

DINNER _____________________

NOTES

____

____

____

____

WEEKLY MEAL PLANNER

MONDAY

BREAKFAST _______________________

LUNCH _______________________

SNACKS _______________________

DINNER _______________________

TUESDAY

BREAKFAST _______________________

LUNCH _______________________

SNACKS _______________________

DINNER _______________________

WEDNESDAY

BREAKFAST _______________________

LUNCH _______________________

SNACKS _______________________

DINNER _______________________

THURSDAY

BREAKFAST _______________________

LUNCH _______________________

SNACKS _______________________

DINNER _______________________

FRIDAY

BREAKFAST _______________________

LUNCH _______________________

SNACKS _______________________

DINNER _______________________

SATURDAY

BREAKFAST _______________________

LUNCH _______________________

SNACKS _______________________

DINNER _______________________

SUNDAY

BREAKFAST _______________________

LUNCH _______________________

SNACKS _______________________

DINNER _______________________

NOTES

____

____

____

____

WEEKLY MEAL PLANNER

MONDAY

BREAKFAST _______________________

LUNCH _______________________

SNACKS _______________________

DINNER _______________________

TUESDAY

BREAKFAST _______________________

LUNCH _______________________

SNACKS _______________________

DINNER _______________________

WEDNESDAY

BREAKFAST _______________________

LUNCH _______________________

SNACKS _______________________

DINNER _______________________

THURSDAY

BREAKFAST _______________________

LUNCH _______________________

SNACKS _______________________

DINNER _______________________

FRIDAY

BREAKFAST _______________________

LUNCH _______________________

SNACKS _______________________

DINNER _______________________

SATURDAY

BREAKFAST _______________________

LUNCH _______________________

SNACKS _______________________

DINNER _______________________

SUNDAY

BREAKFAST _______________________

LUNCH _______________________

SNACKS _______________________

DINNER _______________________

NOTES

____

____

____

____

WEEKLY MEAL PLANNER

MONDAY

BREAKFAST _______________

LUNCH _______________

SNACKS _______________

DINNER _______________

TUESDAY

BREAKFAST _______________

LUNCH _______________

SNACKS _______________

DINNER _______________

WEDNESDAY

BREAKFAST _______________

LUNCH _______________

SNACKS _______________

DINNER _______________

THURSDAY

BREAKFAST _______________

LUNCH _______________

SNACKS _______________

DINNER _______________

FRIDAY

BREAKFAST _______________

LUNCH _______________

SNACKS _______________

DINNER _______________

SATURDAY

BREAKFAST _______________

LUNCH _______________

SNACKS _______________

DINNER _______________

SUNDAY

BREAKFAST _______________

LUNCH _______________

SNACKS _______________

DINNER _______________

NOTES

____

____

____

____

WEEKLY MEAL PLANNER

MONDAY

BREAKFAST _______________________

LUNCH _______________________

SNACKS _______________________

DINNER _______________________

TUESDAY

BREAKFAST _______________________

LUNCH _______________________

SNACKS _______________________

DINNER _______________________

WEDNESDAY

BREAKFAST _______________________

LUNCH _______________________

SNACKS _______________________

DINNER _______________________

THURSDAY

BREAKFAST _______________________

LUNCH _______________________

SNACKS _______________________

DINNER _______________________

FRIDAY

BREAKFAST _______________________

LUNCH _______________________

SNACKS _______________________

DINNER _______________________

SATURDAY

BREAKFAST _______________________

LUNCH _______________________

SNACKS _______________________

DINNER _______________________

SUNDAY

BREAKFAST _______________________

LUNCH _______________________

SNACKS _______________________

DINNER _______________________

NOTES

____

____

____

____

WEEKLY MEAL PLANNER

MONDAY

BREAKFAST ___________________

LUNCH ___________________

SNACKS ___________________

DINNER ___________________

TUESDAY

BREAKFAST ___________________

LUNCH ___________________

SNACKS ___________________

DINNER ___________________

WEDNESDAY

BREAKFAST ___________________

LUNCH ___________________

SNACKS ___________________

DINNER ___________________

THURSDAY

BREAKFAST ___________________

LUNCH ___________________

SNACKS ___________________

DINNER ___________________

FRIDAY

BREAKFAST ___________________

LUNCH ___________________

SNACKS ___________________

DINNER ___________________

SATURDAY

BREAKFAST ___________________

LUNCH ___________________

SNACKS ___________________

DINNER ___________________

SUNDAY

BREAKFAST ___________________

LUNCH ___________________

SNACKS ___________________

DINNER ___________________

NOTES

____

____

____

____

WEEKLY MEAL PLANNER

MONDAY

BREAKFAST ___________________

LUNCH ___________________

SNACKS ___________________

DINNER ___________________

TUESDAY

BREAKFAST ___________________

LUNCH ___________________

SNACKS ___________________

DINNER ___________________

WEDNESDAY

BREAKFAST ___________________

LUNCH ___________________

SNACKS ___________________

DINNER ___________________

THURSDAY

BREAKFAST ___________________

LUNCH ___________________

SNACKS ___________________

DINNER ___________________

FRIDAY

BREAKFAST ___________________

LUNCH ___________________

SNACKS ___________________

DINNER ___________________

SATURDAY

BREAKFAST ___________________

LUNCH ___________________

SNACKS ___________________

DINNER ___________________

SUNDAY

BREAKFAST ___________________

LUNCH ___________________

SNACKS ___________________

DINNER ___________________

NOTES

____

____

____

____

WEEKLY MEAL PLANNER

MONDAY

BREAKFAST _______________________

LUNCH _______________________

SNACKS _______________________

DINNER _______________________

TUESDAY

BREAKFAST _______________________

LUNCH _______________________

SNACKS _______________________

DINNER _______________________

WEDNESDAY

BREAKFAST _______________________

LUNCH _______________________

SNACKS _______________________

DINNER _______________________

THURSDAY

BREAKFAST _______________________

LUNCH _______________________

SNACKS _______________________

DINNER _______________________

FRIDAY

BREAKFAST _______________________

LUNCH _______________________

SNACKS _______________________

DINNER _______________________

SATURDAY

BREAKFAST _______________________

LUNCH _______________________

SNACKS _______________________

DINNER _______________________

SUNDAY

BREAKFAST _______________________

LUNCH _______________________

SNACKS _______________________

DINNER _______________________

NOTES

____

____

____

____

WEEKLY MEAL PLANNER

MONDAY

BREAKFAST ___________________

LUNCH ___________________

SNACKS ___________________

DINNER ___________________

TUESDAY

BREAKFAST ___________________

LUNCH ___________________

SNACKS ___________________

DINNER ___________________

WEDNESDAY

BREAKFAST ___________________

LUNCH ___________________

SNACKS ___________________

DINNER ___________________

THURSDAY

BREAKFAST ___________________

LUNCH ___________________

SNACKS ___________________

DINNER ___________________

FRIDAY

BREAKFAST ___________________

LUNCH ___________________

SNACKS ___________________

DINNER ___________________

SATURDAY

BREAKFAST ___________________

LUNCH ___________________

SNACKS ___________________

DINNER ___________________

SUNDAY

BREAKFAST ___________________

LUNCH ___________________

SNACKS ___________________

DINNER ___________________

NOTES

____

____

____

____

WEEKLY MEAL PLANNER

MONDAY

BREAKFAST __________________

LUNCH __________________

SNACKS __________________

DINNER __________________

TUESDAY

BREAKFAST __________________

LUNCH __________________

SNACKS __________________

DINNER __________________

WEDNESDAY

BREAKFAST __________________

LUNCH __________________

SNACKS __________________

DINNER __________________

THURSDAY

BREAKFAST __________________

LUNCH __________________

SNACKS __________________

DINNER __________________

FRIDAY

BREAKFAST __________________

LUNCH __________________

SNACKS __________________

DINNER __________________

SATURDAY

BREAKFAST __________________

LUNCH __________________

SNACKS __________________

DINNER __________________

SUNDAY

BREAKFAST __________________

LUNCH __________________

SNACKS __________________

DINNER __________________

NOTES

____

____

____

____

WEEKLY MEAL PLANNER

MONDAY

BREAKFAST _______________________

LUNCH _______________________

SNACKS _______________________

DINNER _______________________

TUESDAY

BREAKFAST _______________________

LUNCH _______________________

SNACKS _______________________

DINNER _______________________

WEDNESDAY

BREAKFAST _______________________

LUNCH _______________________

SNACKS _______________________

DINNER _______________________

THURSDAY

BREAKFAST _______________________

LUNCH _______________________

SNACKS _______________________

DINNER _______________________

FRIDAY

BREAKFAST _______________________

LUNCH _______________________

SNACKS _______________________

DINNER _______________________

SATURDAY

BREAKFAST _______________________

LUNCH _______________________

SNACKS _______________________

DINNER _______________________

SUNDAY

BREAKFAST _______________________

LUNCH _______________________

SNACKS _______________________

DINNER _______________________

NOTES

____

____

____

____

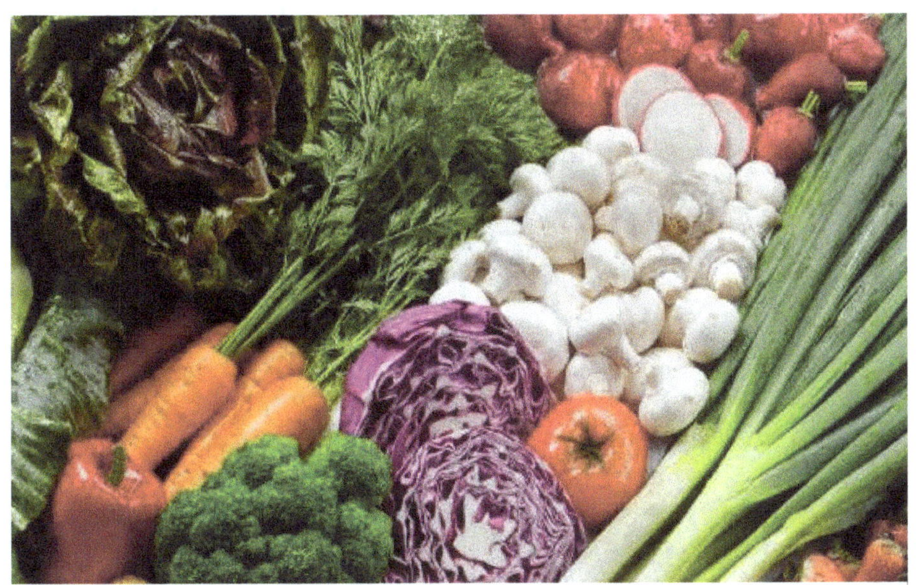

CONCLUSION

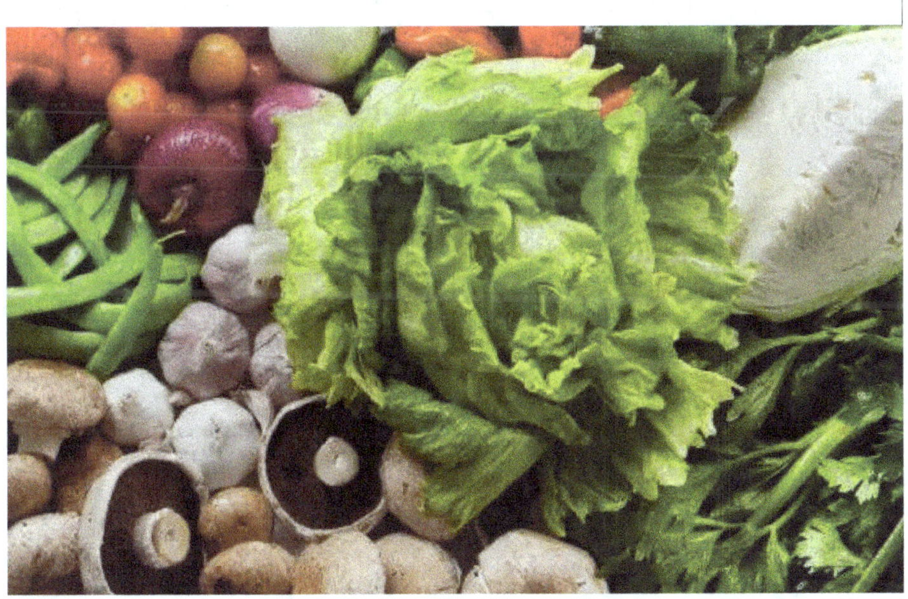

Best wishes! This is the last stop on your trip to a better, more energetic version of yourself. You now have the information and resources necessary to comprehend your metabolism, choose foods wisely, include metabolism-enhancing spices, put quality sleep first, and develop a long-term wellness strategy thanks to this book.

Recall that having a healthy metabolism is only one aspect of the whole. Emotional, mental, and physical health are all components of true well-being. As you proceed on this trip, acknowledge and celebrate all of your accomplishments, no matter how tiny. A healthier you is the result of every decision you make.

Consider this a sustainable lifestyle change rather than a band-aid solution. Finding healthy habits that you can easily incorporate into your everyday routine is the key to long-term success. Try different things, figure out what suits you, and take pleasure in the process of designing a lifestyle that complements your own requirements and tastes.

Recall that achieving and maintaining wellbeing are lifelong endeavors. There will be setbacks, indulgences, and periods of low motivation along the way. Accept these as teaching moments and don't let failure depress you.

Make use of this book as a tool to review important ideas, get motivated, and rekindle your passion for leading a healthy lifestyle.

Celebrate your accomplishments, pay attention to the constructive adjustments you've made, and keep going forward with compassion and empowerment for yourself.

Remember this as you start this thrilling new chapter: you are able to accomplish amazing things. Unlock your full potential for a bright and satisfying life by taking control of your health and adopting a sustainable metabolic lifestyle!